Diagnosis and Management

of Pain Syndromes

BERNARD E. FINNESON, M.D., F.A.C.S.

*Chief of Neurosurgery, Chester, Crozier and
Sacred Heart Hospitals, Pennsylvania;
Neurosurgical Staffs, Albert Einstein Medical
Center and Graduate Hospital, Philadelphia*

Illustrations by Barbara R. Finneson

W. B. SAUNDERS COMPANY
PHILADELPHIA & LONDON

With appreciation to my
friend and associate

DR. HENRY A. SHENKIN

who introduced me to many
of the methods discussed in this monograph.

PREFACE

THIS MONOGRAPH is an attempt to provide a practical and useful guide to the management of the pain problems commonly encountered in practice. Most of the techniques described are widely accepted and no claim is made for original methods or for a "new concept." The material is based on my personal experience in managing pain problems and the procedures are those I have found to be useful. No attempt has been made to describe every known method of treatment. I have purposely limited the scope of the book to the techniques that have worked best for me, endeavoring to impart an orderly and logical approach to the management of a given pain problem. A number of the techniques described fall solely within the discipline of neurosurgery and are not intended as an inducement to those not trained in this field to "try their hand" at an unfamiliar procedure. However, an appreciation of the available operative procedures is helpful to anyone who is involved in the management of pain in order to indicate what can and what cannot be accomplished by neurosurgery.

I am on the neurosurgical staff of the following hospitals and am grateful for their support:

Albert Einstein Medical Center, Philadelphia.
Chester Hospital, Chester.
Crozer Hospital, Chester.
Delaware County Hospital, Drexel Hill.
Episcopal Hospital, Philadelphia.
Graduate Hospital of the University of Pennsylvania, Philadelphia.
Haverford Hospital, Havertown.
Kensington Hospital, Philadelphia.
Sacred Heart Hospital, Chester.
St. Agnes Hospital, Philadelphia.
Taylor Hospital, Ridley Park.
Woman's Hospital of Philadelphia, Philadelphia.

I wish to thank Mrs. Virginia Dougherty, Miss Frances Nettis, and Miss Barbara Quigley for typing and Mrs. Bernice Odom, medical librarian at the Albert Einstein Medical Center, for her assistance. I am indebted to Dr. Stanley Weinstein of Philadelphia for his interesting and invaluable discussions. Dr. Harold Haft has worked in association with me in the management of many of the surgical problems. The elegant illustrations were drawn by my wife whose talent is a source of great personal pride. I want to express my appreciation to the staff of the W. B. Saunders Company for their help and encouragement.

BERNARD E. FINNESON, M.D.

Contents

Diagnosis and Management
of Pain Syndromes

chapter one –

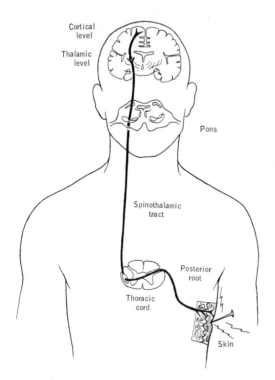

Figure 1. Diagrammatic representation of pain pathways.

Pain and Its Effects

MECHANISMS AND PATHWAYS OF PAIN

The perception of pain is a physiologic process, which involves receptors, conductors, and integrative cerebral mechanisms. All fibers carrying pain impulses enter the spinal cord through the dorsal root ganglions. After entering the cord these impulses are conveyed across the midline to the opposite anterolateral quadrant of the spinal cord where they ascend as fibers of the spinothalamic tract. These fibers travel through the brainstem to the posterolateral and posteromedial nuclei of the thalamus. From the thalamus pain impulses are relayed to the postcentral convolution as well as to the other thalamic nuclei and to the hypothalamus. Awareness of pain appears to take place at the thalamic level, but the cerebral cortex is required for localization and recognition of the quality and degree of pain (Fig. 1).

Pain and Receptor Organs

Until about the beginning of this century touch was considered the fundamental sensation, with warmth and coldness classified as subdivisions of this primary sensation. Pain was regarded as the climax or intensification of touch. However, when exploration of the cutaneous surface of the body was carried out by marking the skin into millimeter squares and carefully testing each square with a small blunt object (pressure), a sharp object (pain), and a warm and a cold object, the existence of touch, pain, heat, and cold spots was revealed. Histologic examination of the skin and other tissues, when correlated with this work, revealed the existence of specific receptors for the various forms of sensation (Fig. 2). Identification of the end-organ for pain was made through the discovery that the weakest perceptible stimuli to the cornea produced pain sensation rather than touch. The only receptors in the cornea are bare nerve endings, and this type of receptor is the only one dis-

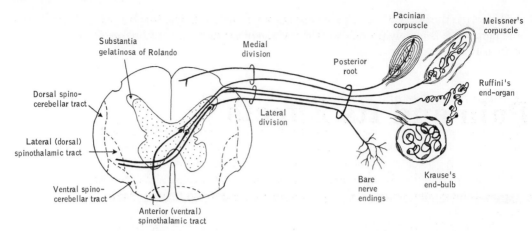

Figure 2. Receptor organs. The various receptor organs and their course into the spinal cord. Note that the pacinian corpuscle and Meissner's corpuscle, which are both tactile or touch end-organs, pass into the cord through the medial division of the dorsal root. Ruffini's end-organ (warmth), Krause's end-bulb (cold), and bare nerve endings (pain) pass through the lateral division of the dorsal root.

tributed widely enough to account for the pain sensitivity of skin, muscle, and viscera.

The sensory end-organs for pain are spread throughout almost all the tissues of the body so that three kinds of pain are recognized: (1) superficial or cutaneous pain; (2) deep pain from muscles, tendons, joints and fascia; and (3) visceral pain.

Adaptation. If a stimulus to a sensory receptor is maintained at a constant intensity the frequency of discharge from this receptor gradually diminishes. This phenomenon is called *adaptation* and the rapidity with which different receptor organs *adapt* varies. The proprioceptors, which are concerned with the automatic maintenance of posture and knowledge of the position of the parts of the body, adapt quite slowly, as is necessary in order to maintain sustained positional attitudes and reflexes. Touch receptors, on the other hand, adapt very rapidly, which is advantageous in order to remain ready to receive new impressions. Pain receptors adapt very little and continue to generate pain impulses for the duration of stimulus. This is consistent with the protective function of pain.

The Adequate Stimulus. For each specific sensory receptor there is one particular stimulus to which the receptor is especially sensitive. This principle is called the "law of adequate stimulus." For example, radiant energy of the visible spectrum is the adequate stimulus to the retina of the eye; sound waves are the adequate stimuli to the ear. However, the phenomenon of the adequate stimulus cannot be applied to the pain receptor since many forms of stimuli are adequate to elicit pain, among them electrical, mechanical, and chemical stimuli and temperature extremes. The chief property common to the various stimuli adequate to excite pain is that they threaten damage to the tissues. Thus, increasing degrees of heat will first stimulate warmth endings, but when the temperature is reached that will damage the skin (50° C.), pain endings are stimulated. The function of the pain sense is mainly protective whereas the other sensory modalities are primarily informative.

Pain and the Peripheral Nerves

The peripheral nerves serve as an intricate conduction system for neural impulses traveling in both directions between the central nervous system and the rest of the body. A peripheral nerve trunk is composed of many nerve fibers bound together by supporting connective tissue. Functionally, three types of fibers may occur in a peripheral nerve, either singly or in combination:

1. Motor fibers, which control voluntary muscular activity by carrying impulses from the central nervous system to skeletal muscles.

2. Sensory fibers, which deliver impulses from the various sensory receptors throughout the body to the central nervous system where they are interpreted as sensations.

3. Autonomic fibers concerned with the control of smooth muscle, glandular activities, and other involuntary bodily functions.

Most charts mapping out the areas of skin innervated by the major cutaneous nerves indicate that each nerve field occupies a discrete and contiguous area, whereas there is usually some overlap between fields (Fig. 3). Because of this overlap a most meticulous sensory examination may reveal little or no area of anesthesia when a small cutaneous nerve is sectioned. Division of a larger cutaneous nerve usually leaves a central zone of total anesthesia surrounded by an intermediate zone of sensory impairment. This intermediate zone is sensitive to painful stimuli and pressure but not to temperature or light touch, and there is some impairment of localization and two-point recognition.

Several days after nerve section the central zone of total anesthesia shrinks circumferentially by extension of the surrounding intermediate zone into it (Fig. 4). At one time this was attributed to rapid regrowth of the interrupted nerve fibers, but the phenomenon occurs before such regeneration could possibly occur. This reduction of the insensible area is due to an ingrowth of fibers from the adjacent peripheral nerve fields, and if the originally interrupted nerve is resectioned, no change is created in the sensory picture. Pain sensation in the intermediate zone is qualitatively altered, for a greater stimulus is required to evoke a pain sensation, but once the threshold is exceeded, the pain is peculiarly strong and unpleasant. This type of "abnormal" pain is also seen when regrowth of the sectioned nerve fibers permits sensation to return to the central anesthetic area.

Pain sensation is carried within the peripheral nerve by two groups of fibers. The so-called "quick" pain is carried by the delta fibers of the "A" group, and a pain perceived somewhat later is carried by the small "C" fibers. This dual projection of pain conduction, a fast and a slow system, explains the phenomenon of double or delayed pain in which the sensation from a brief stimulus is often experienced as two pulses or peaks of pain.

5

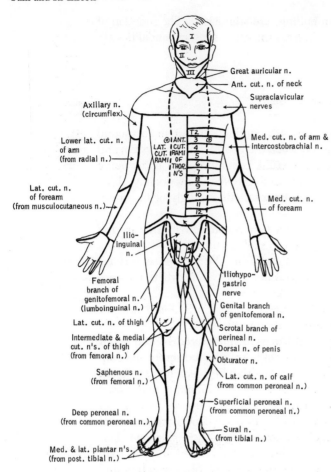

Great auricular n.

Ant. cut. n. of neck

Supraclavicular nerves

Axillary n. (circumflex)

Lower lat. cut. n. of arm (from radial n.)

Med. cut. n. of arm & intercostobrachial n.

Lat. cut. n. of forearm (from musculocutaneous n.)

Med. cut. n. of forearm

Ilio-inguinal n.

Femoral branch of genitofemoral n. (lumboinguinal n.)

Lat. cut. n. of thigh

Intermediate & medial cut. n's. of thigh (from femoral n.)

Saphenous n. (from femoral n.)

Deep peroneal n. (from common peroneal n.)

Med. & lat. plantar n's. (from post. tibial n.)

Iliohypo-gastric nerve

Genital branch of genitofemoral n.

Scrotal branch of perineal n.

Dorsal n. of penis

Obturator n.

Lat. cut. n. of calf (from common peroneal n.)

Superficial peroneal n. (from common peroneal n.)

Sural n. (from tibial n.)

Figure 3. Diagram of peripheral nerve sensory fields.

Since this response is due to the existence of a fast and a slow set of pain fibers, the time between the two pain pulses is greater for stimuli applied to the distal ends of extremities than for proximal portions of the body. For example, a fast and a slow train leaving Philadelphia simultaneously would pass through nearby Trenton fairly close together but would arrive in Boston at significantly different times.

This double pain phenomenon is most apparent when the finger is struck a sharp blow or is brought into contact briefly with a hot object. Immediately after this stimulus, a short, sharp pain is felt that may elicit a reflex withdrawal; this pain disappears quickly. Following this sharp pain, however, there occurs a disagreeable aching pain that lasts a bit longer. If the same stimulus occurs in a more proximal area of the body, the pain is more likely to be felt as a single sensation rather than as two separate pains. In tabes dorsalis, the larger, fast conducting fibers of the "A" group are damaged more than are the "C" fibers, causing a delay of one or two seconds in appreciation of painful stimuli, one of the signs of this disease.

Section of the peripheral nerves may relieve certain types of pain. In senile arthritis of the hip, section of the obturator nerve and the sciatic

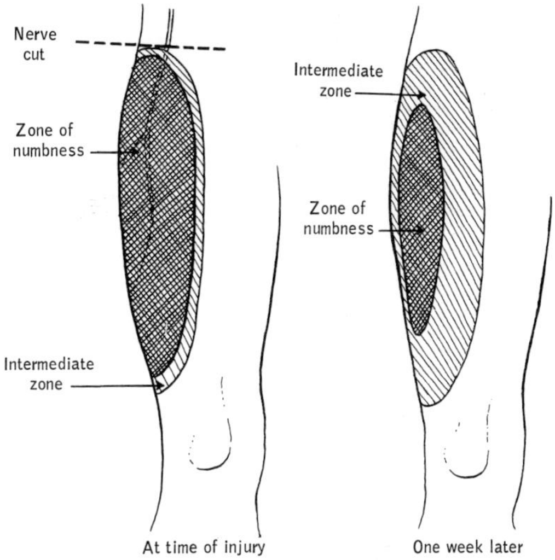

Figure 4. Sensory changes associated with interruption of right lateral femoral cutaneous nerve shortly after onset and one week later.

sensory branch has been beneficial to a significant number of patients. Intractable meralgia paraesthetica may require section of the lateral femoral cutaneous nerve. Supraorbital nerve avulsions have been used widely for management of cases of tic douloureux if the pain is confined to the first division. This procedure is a good example of the tendency for regeneration of peripheral nerves to thwart permanent relief from pain. After supraorbital avulsion, pain usually recurs within several years. On the other hand, a sectioned nerve root of the trigeminal nerve, or any spinal nerve root for that matter, never regenerates and yields permanent relief.

Nerve Roots

The term *nerve root* generally is applied to a bundle of nerve fibers given off from the brainstem or spinal cord that combine to form a cranial or spinal nerve. The spinal nerves consist of an anterior spinal root and a posterior spinal root with its ganglion. The anterior root takes its origin from nerve cells in the anterior and lateral columns of the spinal cord gray matter and passes out of the cord to efferent or motor pathways. The posterior root arises from the medial afferent fibers of the spinal ganglion. This ganglion contains irregularly spherical cells, which give off a unipolar axon that divides into medial and lateral portions. The medial portion is directed to the spinal cord and becomes the posterior root, while the lateral portion is directed peripherally to sensory end-organs of muscles, joints, skin, and viscera (Fig. 5).

The area of skin supplied by a single posterior root is called a dermatome (Fig. 6). To an even greater extent than with peripheral nerves, the dermatomes of adjacent nerve roots overlap so that two and sometimes three roots may supply a single point on the skin. If a single posterior root is sectioned, no anesthesia may result because of this overlap. If, however, several roots

7

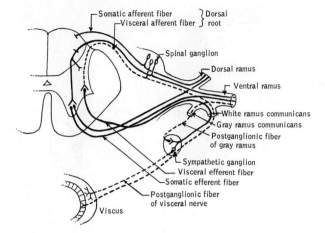

Somatic afferent fiber } Dorsal
Visceral afferent fiber } root

Spinal ganglion

Dorsal ramus

Ventral ramus

White ramus communicans
Gray ramus communicans
Postganglionic fiber
of gray ramus
Sympathetic ganglion
Visceral efferent fiber
Somatic efferent fiber
Postganglionic fiber
of visceral nerve
Viscus

Figure 5. Diagrammatic sketch of motor and sensory nerve roots and their autonomic connections.

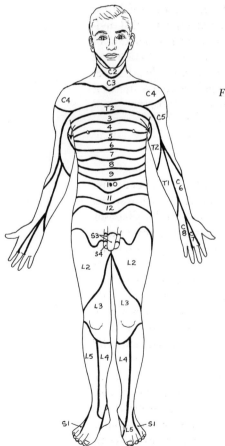

Figure 6. Dermatome map. (After Netter.)

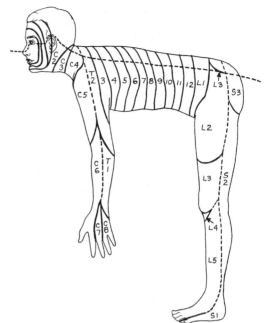

Figure 7. The orderly metameric arrangement of the dermatomes becomes apparent if we visualize man in the quadruped position.

are cut above and below an intact root, this will produce an "island of sensitivity in a sea of anesthesia." The orderly metameric arrangement of the dermatomes becomes apparent if we visualize man in the quadruped position of his far-removed ancestors. In this position the perianal region rather than the feet becomes the terminal portion of the body (Fig. 7). This region, which at one stage of our ontogeny was probably ornamented by a tail, is innervated by the lowermost posterior roots.

Many pain problems are treated by nerve root section or rhizotomy. The standard neurosurgical management of trigeminal neuralgia is retrogasserian rhizotomy in which the sensory roots of the trigeminal nerve are divided. Deep pelvic pain can be relieved by sacral rhizotomy. Bilateral section of the fifth sacral root has been effective for coccydynia. Hip pain has been relieved by section of the posterior lumbar roots. Many painful scars have been relieved by sectioning appropriate sensory roots.

Pain Pathways of the Spinal Cord

Each posterior root breaks up into a fan of rootlets to enter the spinal cord. Upon entering the cord the fibers sort out according to size to form a medial and a lateral division. The medial division contains the large myelinated fibers, which swing across the tip of the posterior horn to enter the posterior columns. The small myelinated fibers, which convey thermal sensibility, and the fine myelinated and unmyelinated fibers, which convey pain, enter the spinal cord through the lateral division and end in the substantia gelatinosa rolandi within one or two segments of the point of entrance. The substantia gelatinosa rolandi is a cell column capping the posterior horn from which second order fibers conduct impulses across the midline in the ventral white commissure and ascend on the opposite side of the cord in the lateral spinothalamic tract.

The ventral spinothalamic tract is a bundle of ascending fibers found in the anterior portion of the cord. It consists of fibers that originate from cells in the posterior gray matter of the opposite side and cross the midline in the anterior white commissure. It is generally stated that the ventral spinothalamic tract is concerned with pain and temperature (Fig. 8), but this functional breakdown is probably not precise, and many physiologists include both the lateral and ventral spinothalamic tracts as subserving the following kinds of sensation: (1) pain from skin, tendons, joints, muscles, and viscera; (2) warmth and cold; (3) itching and muscular fatigue; and (4) pressure and touch (partially spinothalamic).

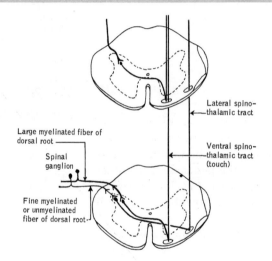

Figure 8.   Formation of the spinothalamic tracts.

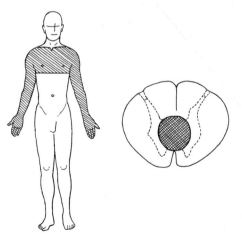

Figure 9.   The sensory changes resulting from a lesion involving the regions of the anterior commissure or central canal within the cervical cord. Shaded area refers to loss of pain and temperature sensation.

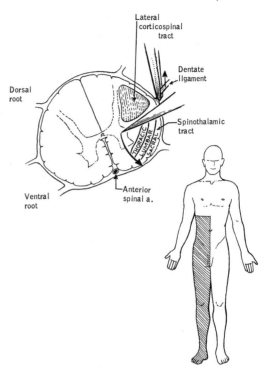

Figure 10. Diagrammatic sketch of cordotomy and the sensory changes produced. Shaded area refers to loss of pain and temperature sensation. Note how position of dentate ligament identifies anterior half of cord and enables surgeon to avoid damage to corticospinal tract.

Any pathologic process in the region of the anterior commissure or central canal—for example, a cyst (syringomyelia) or intramedullary glioma—will interrupt the decussating fibers, producing a clinical syndrome characterized by loss of pain and temperature sensation on both sides of the body at the level of the involved segments; touch and pressure are relatively unaffected (Fig. 9).

A spinothalamic tractotomy, commonly referred to as a cordotomy, is a standard and excellent procedure for the relief of pain. The spinothalamic tract is arranged in a laminated fashion with the fibers of caudal origin placed most superficially and each subsequent layer of fibers representing successively higher levels placed more deeply. This arrangement of fibers makes cordotomy the procedure of choice for pain occurring below the costal margin. Pain above this level may not be affected by the usual 4.5 mm. incision into the cord (Fig. 10).

The Thalamus

The thalamus is a relay station for somatic, visceral, visual, and auditory sensations. This large ovoid structure lying along the wall of the third ventricle and the floor of the lateral ventricle is divided into three parts by a sheath of white matter known as the internal medullary lamina. These portions are redivided into various groups of thalamic nuclei on the basis of morphologic, cytologic, and functional considerations. The function of the

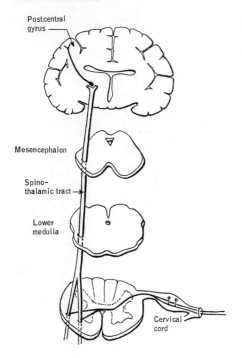

Postcentral
gyrus

Mesencephalon

Spino-
thalamic tract

Lower
medulla

Cervical
cord

Figure 11. Diagram of spinothalamic tracts entering the thalamus from which impulses are relayed to the cerebral cortex.

thalamus is to pass impulses on to the cerebral cortex, and it is presumed that these impulses are integrated by the association nuclei in the thalamus before being relayed. The portion of the thalamus that projects impulses to a specific cortical area receives in return corticothalamic projection fibers from that area, forming a circuit between thalamus and cortex (Fig. 11).

The separate sensory modalities, which are carried in different tracts in the spinal cord and brain stem, partially interdigitate in the thalamus so that modality grouping is largely obliterated. Clinical confirmation of this is demonstrated by the sharp dissociation of the various sensory modalities produced by lesions in the spinal cord but not seen with thalamic lesions.

The thalamus sends fibers to the ipsilateral cerebral cortex, and retrograde degeneration produced by cortical lesions is confined to the thalamus of the same side as the lesion. The so-called *thalamic syndrome* is frequently observed following cerebrovascular accidents that involve the region of the thalamus. This is often described as a burning or aching dysesthesia involving an entire half of the body. The onset of this pain usually occurs several weeks after the "stroke," and discomfort is reported as most intense in the extremities, particularly the hand. Emotional disturbances intensify "thalamic pain," and increased emotional lability with unmotivated laughter or crying is frequently associated with this syndrome.

Utilizing stereotaxic techniques, electrocoagulation of various portions of the thalamus has been carried out for intractable pain and other problems. This procedure is still investigative in nature and cannot yet be considered a standard neurosurgical technique.

The Cerebral Cortex

Sensory mapping of the cerebral cortex has benefited largely from the technical feasibility of performing craniotomies under local anesthesia. The somatosensory cortex is partially located in the region of the postcentral gyrus (Fig. 12). Stimulation of this so-called "sensory strip" near the midline evokes a sensation that seems to come from the foot, while stimulation near the sylvian fissure produces sensations that appear to arise from the face. The sensations are interpreted as coming from the region of the body that is projected upon that cortical area at the site of stimulation. The responses usually reported as a result of cortical stimulation are: tingling, a sense of numbness, or occasionally a sense of movement. Conversely, stimulation of the skin, usually by means of a small brush or a stiff hair, produces cortical action potentials, which can be recorded. This method has been used to "map out" somatocortical representation.

Cerebral lesions confined to the sensory cortex may cause anesthesia during the initial phase of the injury but this is never permanent. Persisting anesthesia is generally thought to reflect extensive subcortical as well as cortical damage, probably affecting projection fibers to the thalamus. Cortical lesions elevate the threshold for all sensations with considerable variation of the various sensory modalities. Pain is usually least modified; pressure and temperature senses are moderately affected. The most severe changes usually occur in light touch and proprioceptive sensation. Preservation of the thalamus is considered sufficient to permit conscious perception of pain sensation. When the sensory cortex of one cerebral hemisphere is completely excised, the resulting sensory impairment is less marked in the face than in the remainder of the body. Resection of various portions of the postcentral convolution has been performed for painful phantom limb and other pain

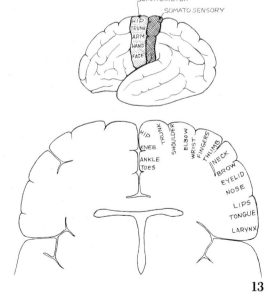

Figure 12. The somatomotor and somatosensory cortex.

13

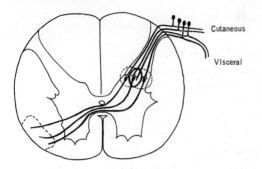

Figure 13. Diagram illustrating one theory of referred pain. Both visceral and cutaneous impulses enter single root and pass to spinothalamic tract. The area of "overlap" shown in the diagram represents a possible "short circuit," which would cause the visceral sensations to be appreciated cutaneously.

problems. The long-term results of these procedures have not been particularly gratifying.

Visceral and Referred Pain

When abdominal surgery is performed under local anesthesia, the visceral organs can be manipulated, incised, cauterized, and crushed without pain if care is taken to avoid traction on the mesentery. This common observation has caused some confusion with regard to visceral sensitivity. Conclusions that the "viscera are insensitive" or that autonomic nerves contain no afferent fibers are refuted by the many painful states associated with diseases involving the abdominal viscera. The principle of the "adequate stimulus" holds true in this area, and adequate stimuli consist of distention, spasm, or chemical irritation. With the exception of the pelvic region, the sympathetic nerves are the principal conductors of visceral pain, while the parasympathetic nerves rarely conduct such impulses. Since the sensory and motor impulses necessary for the regulatory reflexes of the visceral organs are carried only in part by the sympathetic nerves, sympathectomy can be performed for relief of pain without serious disturbance of the denervated organs.

Pain of visceral etiology is frequently appreciated on the surface of the body, and the cutaneous area where such pain is localized may be considerably removed from the involved organ. Although several theories exist to expain this mechanism of referred pain, the cause is not definitely established (Fig. 13). It is known that the dermatomes supplied by the posterior roots, through which the visceral afferent impulses from an organ reach the spinal cord, are involved in referred pain. For example, pain fibers from the heart are carried by the first, second, and third thoracic roots. Since the dermatomes of these roots include the chest wall and the medial aspect of the arm, the classic referred pain pattern of angina pectoris can be predicted.

When visceral pain impulses pass into the spinal cord, they are presumably grouped with deep and cutaneous pain impulses in the anterolateral columns. Section of these tracts (cordotomy) is commonly performed for relief of visceral pain. The thalamic and cortical representations of visceral sensation and pain are not completely understood.

14

PSYCHOLOGY OF PAIN

Pain is a psychobiologic phenomenon with both physical and emotional components. This dual aspect of pain is linked to the distinction between perception of pain and reaction to pain. Perception of pain may be evaluated in terms of quality and intensity, while reaction to pain is manifested by such symptoms as tachycardia, anxiety, fear, panic, and prostration.

Conditioning experiences and emotions may either increase or decrease the reaction to pain, as demonstrated by the howls of pain when a child who is ordered to bed barks his shin on the steps. By contrast, the same injury suffered while climbing to a stadium seat to see a ball game may be unnoticed. The patient harboring malignant disease, whose suffering is always most intense in the gloom of night after all routine activities have ceased and he is alone with his thoughts, is an example of emotional influence that increases the reaction to pain. Often cited to indicate the effect of emotions in decreasing appreciation of pain is the testimony of prize fighters who during the course of a bout may be cruelly battered about and yet not notice any pain during the excitement of the fight. This experience, which is shared by soldiers in combat who often state that their wounds do not become painful until they are evacuated from the dangers of the combat area, is probably only partly due to emotional influences. Initial absence of pain is a common phenomenon accompanying sudden trauma. For example, a bullet wound that shatters the tibia may be appreciated as a heavy but painless blow to the shin. The observation has been made during combat that if a man cries out noisily when wounded, it is likely that the wound is not a severe one. Although high speed projectile wounds are more often mentioned in this connection, stab wounds are often first noticed when blood trickles down the skin.

Under special circumstances the phenomenon of adaptation may come into play and create permanent elevation of pain thresholds. This was the case in a number of Allied prisoners of war subjected to three years of imprisonment and torture by the Japanese during World War II. Some of these survivors had varying degrees of persistent anesthesia, and one had complete insensitivity to all sensations except on the cornea.

A number of papers have described individuals born without a sense of pain. In spite of the lack of this important modality these rare individuals usually are able to cope with the routine problems of daily living and avoid burns and other injuries, which the adult who develops syringomyelia (causing loss of pain and temperature sensations) is prone to incur. Because this condition is extremely uncommon and postmortem confirmation is not available, the site of any possible organic lesion is not known. Some believe that this condition represents a form of sensory agnosia or an aphasia-like inability to formulate an appreciation of pain.

Most psychotic patients do not differ from sane individuals in their reactions to pain. However, many of them complain of severe pain in various portions of their anatomy as a part of their mental illness. On the other hand, some schizophrenic patients have amputated their genitals, fingers, or ears or

15

have extensively mutilated themselves in other ways without expressing a reaction to the pain.

Most well-adjusted individuals who lead active lives experience a number of aches and pains in different parts of their bodies that they ignore. The psychoneurotic person is often prone to seize upon such a nidus of pain and so exaggerate it that the major symptom he eventually produces is so enlarged and distorted it cannot be related to the original pain. The various psychologic mechanisms at work in creating this type of picture vary greatly and should always be considered when the symptoms do not fit into a known clinical pattern.

EVALUATION OF PAIN

The evaluation of pain so that it can be treated adequately is made difficult by its being an entirely subjective phenomenon. It is especially difficult to differentiate organic from psychic factors. The problem is further increased because in most, if not all, patients both factors contribute to the final expression of the pain. Furthermore, the proportion of contributions by the somatic and psychic spheres changes constantly. It is in this area of diagnosis that the "art" of the physician is most severely tested and is least subject to quantitative evaluation and criticism. Estimation of the intensity of pain is likewise difficult for the physician. Nevertheless he must evaluate the intensity in order to determine what therapy is justified for relief of pain. Such questions as the constancy of pain, the interference with performance of duties, and how it affects vital functions, such as sleep, must be answered and clearly evaluated by the examiner.

A careful history is the principal basis for establishing a diagnosis of the pain syndrome and its severity. It often requires considerable time to elicit all the facts that permit the diagnosis of a specific syndrome or to demonstrate that none exists.

An understanding of a patient's personal conception of the workings of his body or of his special medical idiosyncrasies can be instrumental in evaluating the entire clinical picture. A patient with a spinal cord tumor seen some years ago had been hospitalized on two previous occasions for the same complaint of pain radiating into the epigastrium. Because this patient experienced temporary relief of pain following enemas, he was thought to have gastrointestinal disease, and it was not until this man developed long-tract signs with weakness of both lower extremities that disease of the spinal cord was considered. Subsequent questioning revealed that the patient held to an "autointoxication" theory and believed that most body ills were related to chronic constipation.

The patient with a medical history of multiple surgical procedures, frequent hospitalizations, and short "try outs" of a parade of physicians should increase the physician's caution before a diagnosis of organic disease is made. In a large number of pain problems the factor of litigation is present and must be evaluated as a motivating force. As a general rule it is necessary to rest an organic diagnosis upon clear objective changes or on the conformity of the complaints to a known syndrome. Again only a careful and often time-consuming history and examination by an unprejudiced observer will permit a true evaluation of the patient's complaints. Often the behavior of the patient is so bizarre that a firm opinion regarding the existence of any underlying pathologic change cannot be offered. In such instances it is generally wise not to initiate therapy that may cause permanent changes and thus avoid an iatrogenic contribution to the clinical picture.

We will not dwell too long on the obvious importance of a careful physical examination except to note that in managing pain syndromes, some physicians are prone to concentrate exclusively on the patient's symptoms and slur over the physical examination. Many pain problems require special laboratory and x-ray data for differential diagnosis, and it is a common failing to defer these studies in an effort to spare the patient's finances. Any patient with persistent symptoms should have the benefit of complete laboratory and x-ray studies.

chapter two —

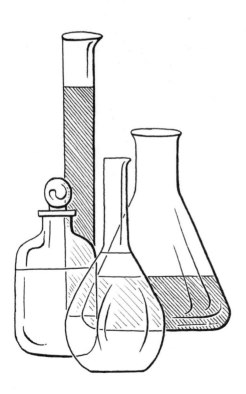

Principles of Treatment

The most important principle in the treatment of pain is avoidance of over-treatment. This pitfall is a great source of potential danger and often tests the physician's critical judgment. The aphorism, "Excess always carries its own retribution," is particularly relevant to the management of pain, for violation of this principle may have unfortunate results.

Still vivid in my memory is the picture presented by an unfortunate man who was a living monument to the hazards of overtreatment. This patient had originally complained of severe pain in the low back and lower extremity for which he was subjected to six myelograms and three lumbar laminectomies. Each successive diagnostic and surgical procedure only served to increase the original pain. The diagnosis of adhesive arachnoiditis of the cauda equina, secondary to the multiple myelograms and surgery, was made and a bilateral cordotomy performed. Following this procedure the patient became paraplegic but continued to complain of his original pain. By this time, the patient was a confirmed narcotic addict and in an effort to control the addiction problem and to alleviate his pain, a prefrontal lobotomy was carried out. A craniotomy wound infection developed, which necessitated removal of the entire frontal bone flap before healing could occur. This extensive bony defect involved the upper half of the forehead and resulted in a particularly unfortunate cosmetic result. The patient then developed severe crossed adductor spasms involving his lower extremities. These were a form of the "mass reflex" involving bladder and bowels so often seen in paraplegia. Because these spasms prevented him from sitting in a wheel chair and in other ways interfered with his general nursing care, a decision was made to section all the lumbar and sacral nerve roots. It was at this stage, when I was a neurosurgery resident, that I first saw the patient and in fact performed this last operative procedure. After the massive rhizotomy, the mass reflex spasms improved but his original pain persisted.

This patient's history revealed that each of his operative procedures was performed by a different surgeon with the exception of the first and third lumbar laminectomies. There is no question that not only were these physicians well intentioned but they were of outstanding professional competence. Obviously each was convinced that the patient's symptoms were nonorganic after he had performed surgery and seen the results. Then another surgeon would be besieged until he was convinced that the patient "deserved another look." The phrase, "We must do something for this suffering patient," has often led to a result worse than the original ailment.

ANALGESICS

Any drug having the property of relieving pain without causing severe impairment of consciousness can be termed an analgesic. This term includes not only those drugs that affect the central nervous system, such as the opiates, but also medications that directly affect the condition giving rise to pain, such as muscle relaxants or vasodilators. Medications that afford specific symptomatic relief will be discussed when the various pain problems requiring these drugs are discussed.

Every "nonspecific" drug that is capable of relieving severe pain has the potential to cause addiction. The addictive properties of these drugs depend on their capacity to create mood changes that allow the patient to accept pain with an attitude bordering on indifference. Pharmacologists have chemically altered these compounds in order to decrease the mood effect, and in doing so they have created medicines with less addictive potentials but that are often less effective in the management of pain.

True drug addiction is mainly a psychologic problem occurring in individuals who are unable to cope with their problems and who use narcotics as a convenient vent. We have performed cordotomies on patients with intractable pain due to carcinoma who required large doses of morphine for prolonged intervals prior to surgery, and after relieving their pain have been gratified that they no longer required narcotics. On the other hand, we have also encountered many previously stable individuals who, after prolonged, intractable pain or because of knowledge regarding their imminent death due to malignant disease, could not be cured of addiction after pain relief had been achieved.

When dealing with a hopeless and painful disease, many physicians deliberately use repeated and ever-increasing doses of narcotics in an effort to make the patient as comfortable as possible. This method is suitable only when life expectancy is limited to less than three months, because ever-worsening emotional problems accompany addiction and the patient becomes so adapted to the drug that he no longer obtains relief of pain. This program of deliberate therapeutic addiction is best carried out in such a way that the patient does not know he is becoming an addict. The physician should not allow the patient to beg for increased amounts of medication but should progressively increase the dosage as required to control pain. At no time should the patient be made fearful that his medication will be terminated, nor is it wise for the physician to behave apprehensively in regard to the large doses required. A program of this nature invariably requires increasing attendance by the physician to avert aberrant behavior and nervousness on the part of the patient.

Opiates

When the milky exudate produced by incising the seed capsule of the poppy plant is dried, it forms a brown, gummy mass called opium. Opium contains numerous alkaloids of which only morphine and codeine have analgesic properties. In addition to the two alkaloids a number of synthetic derivatives of morphine are widely used in the control of pain.

Morphine. Morphine, a central nervous system depressant, acts mainly upon the cerebrum and medulla. The cerebral effects are characterized by a diminution of the usual fears, inhibitions, and worries with an occasional exhilarating feeling of well-being. Loquaciousness and impairment of concentration and logical thinking occur. Hunger is abolished and in some cases is replaced by nausea or vomiting. Apathy may merge into sleep.

The analgesia produced by morphine is quite profound, and use of the drug is indicated for relatively severe visceral and deep traumatic pains. The patient ceases to be disturbed by the pain and may even lose the awareness of pain completely with little impairment of consciousness.

Of prime clinical importance is the respiratory depression produced by the action of morphine on the medulla. Usually this does not become serious unless an overdose is given, but one should always remember that the tolerance for morphine decreases once the original pain has subsided. When the pain is likely to cease abruptly, this type of reaction may occur rather suddenly and require prompt action to prevent tragedy. Some years ago this point was indelibly stamped into the memory of those who were treating a patient with renal colic in the receiving ward. This adult male was in severe distress, and several 15 mg. (¼ grain) doses of morphine only partially alleviated his discomfort, when his pain abruptly subsided, likely as a result of passing the stone. The nurse on duty, who had "taken the trouble" to prepare his next 15 mg. dose, gave him the hypodermic in spite of his announcement that "my pain went away." Shortly thereafter this patient became comatose, unresponsive, cold, clammy, and cyanotic, and his respiratory rate decreased to five a minute. An attending surgeon happened to pass through the accident ward and, promptly assessing the situation, put on a rubber glove and dilated the patient's rectal sphincter to produce pain. The patient's pulse rate instantly increased; within a minute he was semiconscious and in five minutes he was able to communicate.

In addition to increasing pain perception, nalorphine (Nalline) is specific for combating respiratory depression, hypotension, and coma caused by excessive dosage of opiates. The dose of this antagonist to the opiates must of course vary according to the individual reaction. Generally 10 mg. (⅙ grain) is administered intravenously as an initial dose and this may be repeated at 10- or 15-minute intervals. The total dosage should not exceed 40 mg.

Administration and Dosage. Morphine sulfate may be given orally or intravenously, but the commonest route of administration is subcutaneously. The intravenous dosage, 10 mg., should be given slowly, since rapid intravenous administration of morphine may precipitate respiratory depression and may also cause relaxation of the peripheral vessels and a consequent abrupt fall in the blood pressure. The usual dosage range for oral and subcutaneous administration lies between 10 and 15 mg. (⅙ to ¼ grain). If the patient's pain is severe enough to require this powerful analgesic, the half-hour delay in effect following oral dosage is usually too prolonged. Oral administration is useful for chronic pain when the drug is taken at regular intervals before the pain becomes acute.

Side Effects. Nausea and vomiting are more likely to occur when the patient receiving morphine is permitted to ambulate. Frequently this undesirable effect can be controlled by maintaining absolute bed rest and limiting movements of the head from side to side.

Constipation, another undesirable effect of morphine, results from a decrease in contractions of the gastrointestinal tract as well as inattention to the defecation stimulus. The bowel habits of any patient receiving morphine should be determined carefully and appropriate measures taken, including laxatives and enemas, to prevent the development of fecal impaction.

Codeine. Codeine phosphate and codeine sulfate are widely available as 15, 30, and 60 mg. tablets (¼, ½, and 1 grain), which are suitable for hypodermic use when dissolved in water or can be administered orally. As an analgesic, codeine has less than half the effect of morphine and almost no effect on mood. Euphoria and decreased awareness of psychic stimuli are not commonly seen after use of this drug. In the usual doses it does not put the patient to sleep. Codeine is notable in depressing the cough reflex but is much less depressant to the respiratory center and less constipating than morphine.

Codeine is often used in conjunction with antipyretic analgesics (usually aspirin) to augment the effect of the dose. It is used effectively for relief of pains of moderate severity particularly those of a chronic or recurrent nature, such as severe dysmenorrhea or phantom-limb pains, when there is danger of addiction from habitual use. Codeine addiction is rarely reported but can occur if the drug is used for prolonged periods of time. The codeine addict may "graduate" to the more potent drugs and be reported as a morphine or Demerol addict.

Methyldihydromorphinone (Metopon). Metopon is a synthetic derivative of morphine and is available as 3 mg. (½₀ grain) capsules. The minimal effective analgesic dose is 6 mg. or two capsules given orally. The drug produces less sedation and mental confusion and causes less respiratory depression than morphine. The fairly short duration of effect, about two hours, is a disadvantage; the medicine is also more expensive than morphine.

Dihydromorphinone (Dilaudid). This drug, a chemical derivative of morphine, is available in powder, tablets, and ampule solutions for injection. The usual dose ranges between 1 and 4 mg. (¼₄ to ¼₆ grain), which is about one-fifth the dose of morphine, since in equal doses the drug is about five times as potent and as toxic as morphine. Although fully as analgesic as morphine in about one-fifth the dosage, Dilaudid is less constipating and causes less nausea and vomiting. Its action as a respiratory depressant and its addictive liability are about the same as morphine. Like Metopon the drug is more costly than morphine and has a rather short duration of action.

Meperidine (Demerol).   This synthetic drug was originally introduced as a potent analgesic without the danger of addiction. We now know that prolonged use of the drug leads to habituation, but the likelihood of seriously addicting the patient is not so great as with morphine. The analgesic effects of this drug probably lie midway between those of morphine and codeine. Meperidine has a slower onset of effect than morphine, and its action is not so long lasting. Meperidine is less constipating than morphine, and respiratory depression is not usually seen when the recommended dosage is used. However, like all opiates, its use in the presence of intracranial lesions is contraindicated because of the danger of respiratory depression. Nausea and vomiting occur less often than with morphine under similar circumstances. Meperidine is available as an elixir, tablets, and ampules. The usual dose is 100 mg.

Pantopon.   Opium, itself, has properties that make it preferable to morphine or codeine for the treatment of colic or tenesmus accompanying acute diarrhea. However, this insoluble compound is seldom used because it cannot be given hypodermically, and when given orally, the gums it contains delay absorption from the intestine. Pantopon is a mixture of all the alkaloids of opium in the form of their soluble salts, combined in the same proportions as in the natural extract of opium. This preparation can be injected and is available as 10 mg. (⅙ grain) oral tablets and 20 mg. (⅓ grain) ampules. The usual dosage varies between 10 and 20 mg. This drug is more expensive than morphine and has excellent analgesic properties.

Diacetylmorphine (Heroin).   Heroin, a partially synthetic morphine derivitive, is a more potent analgesic than the substance from which it is derived. The usual analgesic dose is 1 to 2 mg. given subcutaneously. It creates marked euphoria; such side effects as nausea, vomiting, and constipation are far less frequent than with morphine. Heroin has created such a serious addiction problem that its importation or manufacture is illegal in the United States.

Salicylates

The two salicylic acid derivatives widely used for their analgesic effects are sodium salicylate and acetylsalicylic acid. Sodium salicylate is a pink, water soluble powder available in 0.3 and 0.6 gm. (5 and 10 grain) tablets and in aqueous solutions for injection containing 1 gm. in 5 cc. The effect of this medication is approximately the same as that of acetylsalicylic acid in most categories of therapeutic activity.

Acetylsalicylic acid is a white powder that is poorly soluble in water and is available in a large variety of tablets and capsules in combination with other drugs. The most widely used form is the 0.3 gm. (5 grain) tablet.

Aspirin is the most popular medication used for minor aches and pains, both as the active ingredient in physicians' prescriptions and in self-medication. About 12 million pounds of salicylates, principally aspirin, are produced annually in the United States.

The analgesic action of the salicylates is markedly less than can be achieved with codeine and is exerted without associated sedative or euphoric effects. The mechanism of the analgesic effect is thought to be some form of central depression but this is uncertain.

The salicylates have maintained their established position against the newer pituitary-adrenal hormone compounds in the treatment of acute rheumatic fever, rheumatoid arthritis, and chronic osteoarthritis. The nature of the antirheumatic action of the salicylates is not known. Some believe that salicylates act by stimulating the anterior pituitary, indirectly stimulating the adrenal cortex to produce cortisone, which creates an antirheumatic effect. Many other theories to explain the antirheumatic action of salicylates have been advanced, including: inhibition of the action of hyaluronidase, inhibition of fibrinolysin, or a direct antiinflammatory effect on blood vessels. At any rate, this amazing drug continues as a sheet anchor in the practice of medicine.

Although the usual dose of 0.6 gm. (10 grains) achieves the maximum elevation of the pain threshold, several times this dosage is necessary when it is used for such conditions as aching joints from arthritis or rheumatic fever. The reason for this seemingly contradictory situation is that the effect of the drug in the latter condition is mainly due to its capacity to reduce inflammation in the involved joint and only incidentally to an elevation of the pain threshold.

Coal-tar Analgesics

Acetanilid, acetophenetidin (phenacetin), and n-acetyl-p-aminophenol are called coal-tar analgesics because they are derived from aniline, which is derived from coal-tar. These drugs are useful as analgesics for minor aches and pains, and like the salicylates they are antipyretics. None of the coal-tar drugs has the antiphlogistic action of the salicylates on acute rheumatic fever.

Both acetanilid and acetophenetidin are converted in the body into n-acetyl-p-aminophenol. It is thought that this drug elevates the pain perception threshold at some point between the thalamus and cortex. Sedative or hypnotic effects are not associated with the action of this drug.

N-acetyl-p-aminophenol is widely available only as a solution (Tylenol) containing 120 mg. per 5 cc. for oral administration. It is usually prescribed for infants and children at four-hour intervals. The dosage scale according to age is: 2.5 cc., less than 12 months of age; 5 cc., one to four years; and 5 to 10 cc., four to six years.

Both acetanilid and acetophenetidin must be taken in the form of effervescent powder or as tablets or capsules because they are too poorly soluble to prescribe in solution. The average adult dose of acetanilid is 200 mg. (3 grains) and of acetophenetidin, 300 mg. (5 grains). Each may be taken at three-hour intervals, but it is inadvisable to prescribe more than six such successive doses without a drugless interval because the accumulation of these agents in the body is toxic. Signs of drug toxicity include confusion, dyspnea, clammy sweat, cold extremities, subnormal temperature, rapid weak pulse, and cyanosis.

There are numerous proprietary preparations that include one of the coal-tar analgesics in combination with other drugs, such as caffeine and aspirin (Empirin compound) or barbiturates. Many proprietary powders that effervesce when placed in water contain a coal-tar analgesic.

PLACEBOS

I was once called in consultation to see a patient with a pain problem and, upon inquiring about the efficacy of placebos on the patient's pain, was told by the attending physician that this type of "deception" was never prac-iced on his patients. The physician who made this statement was extremely able and conscientious and, because of his obvious sincerity and concern for the health of his patients, enjoyed their trust and confidence to an un-usual degree. It is certain that whatever medications he prescribed, the re-sults were frequently augmented by a placebo effect based on his splendid personality. Viewed realistically, many types of treatment other than the traditional capsule filled with lactose can create the placebo effect, since this is based upon trust in the physician and faith in medicine generally. We have all seen patients whose intractable pain from malignant disease was temporarily relieved by an injection of sterile water. This is completely in accordance with our present understanding of psychosomatic medicine and the interrelationships of the mind and somatic illness. It has been shown that placebos can actually cause changes in laboratory data, such as the sedimentation rate, carbon dioxide combining power, and the white blood cell count. The faith of the prescribing physician in a drug may have a def-inite effect on its action.

Knowledge of the placebo effect has led to the use of the "double blind" method of testing drugs in which the physician as well as the patient is unaware of whether the drug being administered is a placebo or the medi-cation being tested. Just as many executives maintain that the best sales-men are not necessarily the brightest men but usually those who are the most enthusiastic about the product, so may the physician who actually be-lieves in the curative properties of the drug he is giving create a greater effect than the doctor who is realistically uncertain about the merits of the medicine prescribed. In addition to drugs, physical measures including dia-thermy and massage create a positive psychologic effect, which is the basis for the use of these techniques by many healing cults, such as chiropractic and naturopathy.

Probably surgery has the most potent placebo effect that can be exer-cised in medicine. The detailed preliminaries, the rendering unconscious via anesthesia, the removal or the manipulation of vital organs within the body all create an almost mystic and profound emotional effect on the patient. This effect, of course, varies greatly from patient to patient, but in evaluat-ing the results of any large series of surgical procedures this placebo effect must certainly be considered. A well-known physician, an outstanding pio-neer in the field of neurosurgery, when faced with a problem case of low back pain that he believed to be nonorganic in etiology, occasionally re-sorted to having the patient prepared and anesthetized for laminectomy and

25

merely made the skin incision, which he then promptly sutured. Several cases were cured by this management.

ANALGESIC BLOCK

Indications

Relief of Pain. Most analgesic blocks are used to obtain symptomatic relief of severe pain. The analgesia created by injection of local anesthesia, in addition to affording temporary relief of pain, permits the use of other methods of treatment that would otherwise be excessively painful. For example, manipulation of the painful shoulder is more readily performed following a block, which creates analgesia in the area. Occasionally analgesic blocks create a prolonged beneficial effect beyond the effective duration of the agent injected. This is thought to be due to interruption of reflexes that take part in causing sustained pain.

Diagnosis. A number of pain syndromes can be identified with the aid of diagnostic blocks. For example, in differentiating the various types of facial pain caused by involvement of the fifth, ninth, or tenth cranial nerves, temporary blocks of these nerves may be helpful in diagnosing a typical form of these syndromes.

Prognosis. When permanent interruption of a nerve is contemplated, a temporary block may be helpful in determining the benefit to be obtained from such proposed surgery.

Technique

In order to obtain optimal results with any analgesic block, one should be prepared to spend enough time to assure careful and measured placement of the needle. Not only should the physician be familiar with the procedure but he must also be cognizant of the various contraindications and complications of each block that he performs.

Preparation of the Patient. A variable degree of discomfort occurs during the performance of almost any block, and the use of preliminary medications may be of help, not only in reducing discomfort but in securing the patient's cooperation during the procedure. When the correct position of the needle is signaled by paresthesia, the patient is told what to expect and is instructed to inform the physician as soon as this sensation is appreciated.

Asepsis. The injection site is cleansed with alcohol or other antiseptic solutions. Sterile gloves are worn during the performance of the block. Before preparing the skin with antiseptic solution it is advisable to identify the landmarks. Sterile towels draping the field are best placed in such a fashion that the landmarks are not obscured.

Use of the Needle. Before using the needle, one should look carefully for burrs on the point, and the patency of the lumen should be tested by injecting solution through the needle.

In attempting to block a nerve many beginners make the mistake of thrusting it through tissue in rapid stabbing movements similar to the technique used to enter a blood vessel. The correct method is to advance slowly and carefully so that as soon as the nerve is contacted the position of the needle can be maintained.

Equipment

A special tray containing all the essentials necessary to perform analgesic blocks is an expediency that does away with the annoying task of collecting the various bits of equipment each time a block is performed. The tray should include two containers: one for antiseptic and the other for the local anesthetic solution. Several squares of gauze are used for preparing the skin with antiseptic and three towels are used to drape the sterile field. A "three-ring" 10 cc. syringe with a lock tip is the most convenient type for general use, and a 2 cc. syringe is included for alcohol blocks. A 2 cm., 25-gauge hypodermic needle is used for the intradermal wheal. A variety of needles for deeper injections should include two 20-gauge, 15 cm.; two 20-gauge, 10 cm.; and two 22-gauge, 10 cm. (all these needles should be of the lumbar puncture type with fitted stylets). A ruler calibrated in inches and centimeters as well as several depth markers made of small rubber squares completes the tray.

Drugs Used for Analgesic Blocks

Local anesthetics affect sensory nerve fibers more readily than motor fibers, and this can be demonstrated by infiltrating a mixed (motor and sensory) nerve and producing complete anesthesia with little or no discernible motor weakness. In addition to pain fibers, the small unmyelinated or thinly myelinated fibers carrying sympathetic impulses are quite susceptible to the action of local anesthetics.

Procaine. Procaine is the most commonly used local anesthetic. It establishes analgesia in three to ten minutes, depending on the concentration of the drug and the size of the nerve to be blocked. The duration of anesthesia is usually less than one hour. The amount of drug used should never exceed 15 mg. per kilogram of body weight in adults and 5 mg. per kilogram of body weight in children. A clinically effective level of surface analgesia of mucous membranes cannot be obtained by topical application of the usual concentration of this drug.

Lidocaine (Xylocaine). Lidocaine has several distinct advantages over procaine and I consider it the local anesthetic of choice. It acts more promptly and can be used with equal effectiveness in one-half the concentration of procaine. The duration of effect is about twice that of procaine —about two hours. The toxicity of this drug is about the same as procaine for the same concentrations. Another advantage possessed by this drug is the satisfactory surface analgesia obtained when it is applied topically to mucous membranes.

27

Pontocaine, Metycaine, Nupercaine, and Intracaine are other local anesthetic agents in wide use. I have had no personal experience with them, but in clinics where these various drugs are employed the reports are generally favorable.

Cocaine. Cocaine is used only for topical anesthesia and is absolutely contraindicated in infiltration anesthesia because of its great toxicity. It is used in a 4 per cent concentration for topical use and in a 10 per cent concentration in an atomizer for topical spray. No more than 100 to 150 mg. of cocaine should be used at one time. Toxic doses of cocaine cause central nervous system depression, starting with the cortex, progressing to the medulla, and leading to myocardial depression. This may create hypotension and complete cardiovascular collapse.

The Supplementary Use of Epinephrine. All the drugs used for local anesthesia are vasodilators. The addition of a vasoconstrictor (epinephrine) to these drugs not only prolongs the effect of anesthesia by creating local vasoconstriction and allowing the anesthetic agent to remain in contact with the tissues for a longer time but, by decreasing the rate of absorption into the general circulation, prevents the anesthetic from reaching a toxic blood level. The optimum amount of epinephrine is that which will result in a 1 to 200,000 final concentration after it is added to the local anesthetic. Thus, 1 cc. of a 1 to 1000 solution (1 mg.) of epinephrine is added to each 200 cc. of anesthetic solution or 0.1 cc. of 1 to 1000 epinephrine for each 20 cc. of anesthetic solution.

Toxic Reactions

Drug Idiosyncracy. True hypersensitivity to a local anesthetic or drug idiosyncracy is very rare but it does occur. Because such reactions may occur with minute doses, sometimes merely a skin wheal, they are almost impossible to avoid. The reaction consists of sudden cardiovascular and respiratory collapse, which may be followed rapidly by cardiac arrest and death.

Treatment. The patient is placed immediately in the head-down position, and if respirations have ceased, artificial respiration and oxygen are administered. If oxygen is not immediately available, artificial respiration is performed by mouth-to-mouth breathing. Intravenous administration of vasopressor drugs is instituted to combat the circulatory collapse. If cardiac arrest occurs, cardiac massage is performed immediately.

Toxicity Due to Overdosage. Most undesirable reactions occurring with the use of local anesthetics are due to lapses in technique that permit excessive concentrations of local anesthetics to accumulate in the systemic circulation. The errors leading to this type of reaction are inadvertent injection into a blood vessel or the use of excessive quantities of anesthetic.

The severity of this type of reaction depends on the quantities of anesthetic agent in the systemic circulation and varies from lightheadedness and vertigo to drowsiness, confusion, and muscular twitching, which may progress to convulsions.

Treatment. Reactions characterized by confusion and muscular twitching require immediate treatment to prevent hypoxia and to inhibit convulsions. Oxygen is administered and the airway maintained by any means necessary. A rapidly acting intravenous barbiturate (Pentathol) is administered as soon as muscular twitchings are noted in an effort to prevent frank convulsions. Sufficient barbiturate is given to control the muscular activity.

If a very great concentration of the anesthetic agent finds its way into the systemic circulation, severe circulatory collapse occurs with coma, hypotension, and bradycardia. When this occurs, administration of barbiturate is contraindicated because it would aggravate the preexisting central nervous system depression. Treatment in this case consists of management of shock with vasopressors and use of the head-down position as well as adequate aeration with oxygen, artificial respiration, and maintenance of a proper airway.

chapter three —

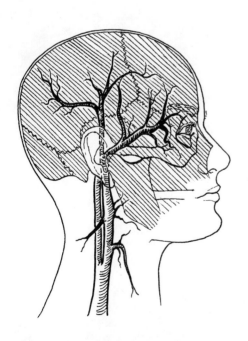

Headache

Headache is probably the most common symptom in medicine. It is also one of the most confusing, because although it usually occurs in the absence of organic changes, it may be a manifestation of serious disease.

Wolff and his associates have studied the various mechanisms involved in headache from both physiologic and psychologic points of view. To ascertain the pain-sensitive structures of the head, Wolff and Ray studied 45 patients who underwent cranial surgery under local anesthesia. They found that stimulation of, pressure on, or traction on the following produced pain:

1. All tissues covering the cranium.
2. The large intracranial venous sinuses.
3. The fifth, ninth, and tenth cranial nerves.
4. The upper cervical nerves.
5. The large arteries at the base of the brain.
6. The large dural arteries.
7. The dura mater at the base of the skull.

Dilatation or contraction of the walls of blood vessels also caused pain.

With this information it is possible to explain headache of somatic origin on the basis of alterations in one or more of these structures. Thus, the headaches associated with brain tumor, with alterations in intracranial pressure, with hypertension, and even migraine can be better understood and delineated. On the other hand, the headache of psychogenic origin cannot yet be explained on a clear anatomicophysiologic basis. It is conceivable, and indeed probable, that as understanding of the problem grows, a number of entities will be separated from the group of "tension headaches" and assigned a primary anatomic or a physiologic classification. Indeed, in time psychosomatic mechanisms may well be determined for the tension state itself, permitting a more physiologic approach to its treatment than is now available.

The occasional mild headache that almost every adult has appreciated at some time does not present much of a problem. It is usually related to

31

such causes as eyestrain, systemic illness, fatigue, or dietary or alcoholic excesses, and even if the etiology is uncertain because of the mild short-lived nature of the symptoms, a few aspirin tablets suffice for therapy. On the other hand, the chronic or repeatedly recurring headache presents a great challenge with regard to diagnosis and management. All patients with persistent headaches that do not respond to therapy should, as part of their medical management, be hospitalized for complete studies, which should include lumbar puncture, x-ray of the skull, and electroencephalography.

MIGRAINE

Definition

Migraine is generally defined as an episodic headache, usually unilateral, that is associated with nausea. We believe that the term migraine should be reserved for a specific syndrome, the organic basis for which can be reasonably presumed. Limited in this manner, the cases to which the term migraine can be applied are relatively few; many diagnosed as "migraine" are simply tension headaches.

Symptoms and Signs

It is widely accepted that the migrainous syndrome consists of four components: headache, gastrointestinal disturbances (particularly nausea and vomiting), visual disturbances (especially scintillating scotoma), and a family history of headaches. Any of these components may predominate, and one or more may be absent. The classic migraine occurs in an individual in relatively good health who develops periodic, incapacitating headaches often preceded by visual and vasomotor disturbances with nausea and vomiting occurring during the peak or culminating the attack. Migraine sufferers characteristically are driving, ambitious, and obsessive. They are generally professionals, executives, or housewives rather than laborers or open air workers. A large percentage of these patients have a definite family history of migraine. Although considerable variation occurs from patient to patient, the individual sufferer usually reports a standard pattern in his own recurrent attacks. The pain is frequently hemicranial, but it may be localized to a fairly small area, or it may extend into the face, neck, or shoulders; or indeed it may be generalized and involve the entire head. The most common description of the pain is throbbing, but pressure or a sensation of fullness within the skull or of rhythmic, hammer-like blows to the head are also described.

Symptoms preceding the attack may have been unnoticed by the patient and only direct questioning will elicit them. They usually consist of a change in mood. Hours or days before there may have been a sense of malaise, diminished energy, irritability, somnolence, or emotional depression. Occasionally, immediately preceding a migraine, the patient may feel unusually happy and comfortable with a sense of well-being, euphoria, and mental lucidity.

The prodromal symptoms occur in about 10 per cent of migraine sufferers and are due to an initial cerebral vasoconstriction lasting a few minutes to an hour. Most commonly the prodrome consists of eye signs, such as scintillating scotomata or homonymous hemianopsia. Occasionally ophthalmoplegia is reported. Less frequently unilateral paresthesia, paresis, or aphasia occurs.

The headache may be divided into two stages. The initial headache starts slowly, is throbbing and pulsating in character, and is usually hemicranial. It may then spread to other areas. The headache starts on the same side in 90 per cent of attacks and is usually accompanied by nausea and frequently by vomiting. It is believed that the pain is due to vasodilatation of extracerebral vessels.

The entire attack may last several hours to several days. By contrast with tension headache, there is generally no interference with sleep, which frequently helps decrease the headache.

Treatment

Psychotherapy.   Almost any type of treatment that is administered with enthusiasm by the physician may achieve a psychologic effect and diminish the frequency and intensity of attacks for a limited time.

The chief problem is the obsessive nature of the migraine patient, who is intolerant both to the less exacting performance of his associates and to his own personal failings. The fierce ambition and great energy that these patients frequently possess may run counter to an orderly existence, and, therefore, if the physician can bring insight into the problem, the severity and frequency of the attacks may be reduced.

In our experience, the use of psychoanalysis has proved disappointing. We believe that a more superficial approach is of greater benefit and that the physician must point out as clearly as possible the price the patient must pay if he wishes to continue his symptom-producing activities. Frequently the migraine patient is unable to solve his own problem without assistance and responds best to specific suggestions. This may indicate why psychoanalysis with its passive, nondirective approach is rarely beneficial. Most patients are not completely aware of the specific factors causing their symptoms or in many cases refuse to admit their existence. For this reason, rather than questioning them about stress situations, the physician should attempt to obtain a detailed account of daily routine that will allow him to estimate the emotional and physical demands made upon the patient. In regulating the patient's routine to avoid overwork, fatigue, and emotional strain it is important to preserve his self-respect by indicating that following such a course does not make one a "quitter," but that on the contrary increased effectiveness may well result from greater work satisfaction.

Unless the physician is willing to spend an adequate amount of time in dealing with the psychologic aspects of migraine, little can be accomplished in this sphere. We have found tranquilizer medication of some benefit during the transition period when the patient is making efforts to reduce emotional tension by changes in his routine.

According to the needs of the individual patient, other mechanisms for furthering relaxation are indicated. In some, physical exercise in the form of golf or tennis is advisable, while in others, routine rest periods, preferably taken lying down on a bed or a couch, are recommended. A type of "hydrotherapy" in which the patient relaxes in a warm tub for a half hour daily before dinner is frequently effective in reducing tension.

The physician should be cautious about suggesting drastic changes. One of our patients had been advised to retire from his job because of severe migraine only to have his headaches worsen. When he returned to his occupation and regulated his existence to minimize "tension peaks," his work became a therapeutically valuable emotional outlet and his headaches diminished. Another common misconception is to regard as advantageous work involving physical rather than mental effort. Many a farmer, concerned about his crop, can be under considerably more tension than the so-called "high strung" business man who leads a sensibly regulated life.

Drugs. The low intensity migraine headache occasionally can be treated by the oral administration of aspirin (0.3 to 0.6 gm.), supplemented by codeine sulfate (30 to 60 mg.) if the pain is of greater intensity. If codeine causes nausea or constipation, 32 or 65 mg. of dextropropoxyphene (Darvon) may be used. In unusual cases it is necessary to use morphine sulfate (15 mg.) to terminate an extremely severe headache. This drug should not be used until all others fail, and, in our experience, once adequate management of the case is accomplished, a powerful narcotic of this nature is never required routinely.

Ergotamine tartrate is a vasoconstrictor that reduces the pain-producing vasodilatation of the cranial arteries during the migraine attack. This drug should not be used in patients with severe arteriosclerosis, coronary heart disease, Raynaud's syndrome, Buerger's disease, or infectious states or in pregnant patients. Nausea, vomiting, numbness and tingling of the extremities, muscular stiffness of the thighs and posterior cervical muscles, and exhaustion are common side effects of the drug. These symptoms usually persist less than 24 hours; if these symptoms last longer, the drug should not be used again.

Ergotism resulting from the use of this drug in migraine is almost unheard of. The syndrome consists of severe vomiting followed by swelling and cyanosis of the feet with disappearance of peripheral pulses. This may eventually progress to gangrene.

Ergotamine tartrate can be administered intramuscularly, intravenously, orally, or sublingually or inhaled in an aerosol vehicle. Intramuscular administration of a dose of 0.25 to 0.50 mg. is the most effective method. This dose may be repeated in two hours if symptoms are not relieved, but no more than 1 mg. should be administered in 24 hours. This injection is best given by the physician so that the patient's routine can be regulated properly, although some doctors have instructed their patients to give themselves the intramuscular injections. We consider this an error in management because of the possibility of excessive dosage as well as impairment of the physician's firm control in the medical management of the case. The migraine patient should not be made to feel that there is a lack of interest on the part of the doctor. The oral route has all the disadvantages of self-injection in addition to being less effective. There is also the added confusion caused by vomiting following the oral intake of the drug, which creates uncertainty regarding the amount of medication absorbed if an intramuscular injection is contemplated subsequently. The oral or sublingual dosage is 5 mg. at the onset of the headache followed by 2 mg. each hour until the headache ceases or a total of 10 mg. has been ingested. The recently developed aerosol suspension of ergotamine tartrate is designed for oral inhalation of a metered dose of 0.36 mg. This method is less effective than intramuscular administration but superior to the oral preparations.

If relief of symptoms is achieved with the use of ergotamine, the patient may wish to resume his activities promptly. The physician should make clear to the patient that the basis of his symptoms is the protest made by his body against the emotional and physical demands created by the routine he wishes to continue. He must rest undisturbed for at least two hours after the attack subsides. If necessary, 1.5 gr. of Seconal can be used to produce sleep, although frequently the natural lethargy following a migraine attack is sufficient to promote sleep.

Because caffeine, when given orally, is reported to act as a vasoconstrictor, 100 mg. of this drug has been combined with 1 mg. of ergotamine and marketed as Cafergot. The usual dosage is two tablets at the onset of headache or, if present, during the aura (prodromal symptoms) of the migraine attack, followed by one tablet at half-hour intervals until relief occurs (a maximum of six tablets). This combination is also supplied in suppository form (containing 2 mg. of ergotamine tartrate and 100 mg. of caffeine) for use when severe vomiting is present. One suppository is used as early as possible in the attack, followed by a second suppository in one hour, if needed; no more than two suppositories should be used.

If nausea and vomiting present a problem in the administration of ergotamine, the use of atropine sulfate (0.4 mg.) with each dose may be helpful.

Some patients who are unable to tolerate ergotamine may be benefited by dihydroergotamine (D.H.E. 45), which has fewer and milder side effects. This drug is given intramuscularly in a 1 mg. dose, which may be repeated in one hour. It is not so effective as ergotamine tartrate.

When the migraine is continuous and remains severe ("status migrainous"), it frequently is necessary to use hypnotic doses of barbiturates in addition to ergot. We insist on hospitalizing such a patient because of the many dangers and complications that may occur when a deeply narcotized patient is unattended by medical and nursing personnel. In addition, these patients frequently present a moderate dehydration problem owing to vomiting and inadequate fluid intake, which is best managed by intravenous infusions.

Other Procedures. Understanding of the cerebral vascular changes (arterial dilatation) producing migraine has renewed interest in a surgical treatment for this syndrome. Since the most direct method of eliminating arterial dilatation is interruption of the vessel, a number of arteries in the

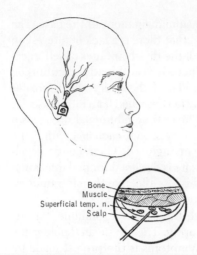

Bone
Muscle
Superficial temp. n.
Scalp

Figure 14. Infiltration of the superficial temporal artery. The anesthetic agent should be injected so that the entire circumference of the involved artery is contacted.

neck and head have been ligated for this disease. This approach is theoretically sound, and in fact many migraine headaches have been diminished and occasionally interrupted by firm pressure on the carotid pulse in the neck or the temporal pulse in the scalp. From a practical standpoint arterial ligation has not proved uniformly successful, even if improvement initially occurs, because of the tendency for collateral vessels to enlarge and the original vascular status to recur. On the other hand, useful results lasting many years have been achieved occasionally with surgery in patients who had not responded to medical management.

Local infiltration of the superficial temporal artery and other superficial scalp vessels can be used as a prognostic block in determining the effectiveness of excision of segments of these vessels (Fig. 14). The anesthetic agent should be injected so that the entire circumference of the involved artery is contacted. Ligation of the superficial temporal artery is a relatively minor procedure that can be done under local anesthesia (Fig. 15). Some patients have responded to ligation of the external carotid artery in the neck alone or in combination with removal of a length of superficial temporal artery. Ligation of the middle meningeal artery is a major procedure requiring a temporal craniectomy for exposure of the vessel. Such a procedure should be contemplated only if external carotid ligation has produced improvement for at least six months, the subsequent formation of a collateral circulation causing the middle meningeal to regain its original capacity to dilate. Another indication for ligation of the middle meningeal artery is localization of the pain in the low temporal region immediately above the zygoma.

A number of patients with intractable migraine have been benefited by interruption of the trigeminal nerve. This procedure should only be used when the pain is located in an area innervated by the fifth cranial nerve. Because it is a relatively minor procedure, supraorbital avulsion of the first division is occasionally performed when the headache is confined to the frontal area. These procedures, unfortunately, are rarely successful. When interruption of the trigeminal nerve is indicated, the procedure of choice is

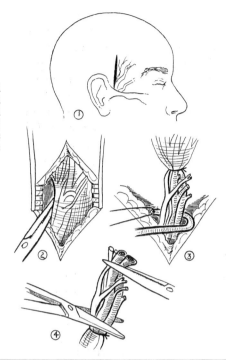

Figure 15. Ligation of superficial temporal artery. (1) Incision made anterior to ear and above the zygoma. (2) Branches of superficial temporal artery and nerves dissected out. (3) Mass ligature used to ligate bundle of arteries and nerves (using aneurysm needle to pass ligature). (4) Segment of bundle excised.

the classic trigeminal rhizotomy through the temporal approach. Before undertaking such surgery, which provides permanent anesthesia, alcohol blocks to peripheral branches should be used to determine the effect, if any, of anesthesia, which will persist for at least several months.

HISTAMINE CEPHALGIA

Definition

Histamine cephalgia is a unilateral headache characterized by high intensity, burning pain. The pain usually begins suddenly, lasts less than an hour, and ceases as abruptly as it began.

Symptoms and Signs

This syndrome, which was first delineated by Horton, almost always occurs in males, usually developing after the age of 40. The pain is always excruciating, occasionally is described as boring, and follows the distribution of the external carotid artery, involving the eye, temporal area, neck, and face. It sometimes extends into the shoulder on the involved side. The attacks may occur several hours after the patient has gone to sleep, frequently awakening him; at times the pain is so severe that the patient finds himself sitting up in bed or even jumps out of bed before he is completely awake.

37

During and following the attack, tenderness is frequently present in the painful region, particularly over the distribution of the external carotid artery. Vasomotor phenomena are constant and may include lacrimation, rhinorrhea, swelling of the temporal vessels, and erythema or increased skin temperature in the area of the pain. The frequency of the attacks may increase until they occur every few hours for prolonged periods of time.

In certain respects the condition resembles migraine, but the following important features permit a differentiation: Histamine cephalgia occurs predominantly in males over 40 years of age. The attacks have a sudden onset, a short duration, and an abrupt subsidence. They are not preceded by an aura, and cerebral phenomena, such as hemianesthesia, visual scotoma, and mood changes, are absent as are nausea and vomiting.

Pathophysiology

Many patients who are susceptible to this type of headache have a history of allergy, and in some cases a specific relationship to food or some other allergic substance can be established. The subcutaneous injection of 0.35 mg. of histamine diphosphate usually precipitates an attack in the patient suffering from histamine cephalgia. Although this medication may produce an immediate generalized headache of short duration in the normal individual, the pain it causes in the patient with histamine cephalgia is unilateral and in all respects identical to the spontaneous attacks. Both the spontaneous and the induced attacks may be terminated by intravenous administration of 1 cc. of a 1 to 400,000 solution of epinephrine.

Treatment

An increase in the amplitude of arterial pulsations is common to both histamine cephalgia and migraine. However, ergotamine is not so uniformly successful in the management of this symptom as it is with migraine, probably because the lack of aura, the rapidity of onset, and the relatively short duration of the attack give the medication scant time to create an effect before the pain has subsided spontaneously. Because of these factors, prevention of subsequent attacks is the chief objective of treatment by means of histamine desensitization. This can be accomplished by giving histamine diphosphate subcutaneously twice daily, starting with 0.02 mg. and increasing the dosage by 0.02 mg. daily up to 0.4 mg. twice daily. After 30 days the frequency of the dose is gradually decreased. Marked flushing is anticipated, but if severe headaches are caused by this medication the dosage is reduced accordingly. This drug can also be given intravenously, using 2.75 mg. of histamine diphosphate in 250 cc. of physiologic saline daily, allowing the infusion to run at a rate that allows the patient to remain barely flushed.

We have had little success with the use of antihistaminics for histamine cephalgia. Benadryl (50 mg.) and Pyribenzamine (25 mg.) are reported to give prompt relief of symptoms. In our experience the secondary sudomotor and vasomotor phenomena are frequently alleviated with little or no effect on the headache.

MUSCLE TENSION HEADACHE

Definition

Although the term *tension headache* is sometimes used interchangeably with *psychogenic headache*, we refer specifically to headache resulting from sustained contractions of the skeletal muscles of the head and neck. Of course, the most common cause of such sustained muscle contraction is anxiety and emotional tension, but occasionally other stimuli can produce the same reaction. Muscle tension may be secondary to other types of headaches, such as migraine. Some individuals develop muscle tension headache after exposure to cold that causes them to shiver. We recently treated a patient who was a native of Philadelphia and was quite inured to the "Eastern winters." Following a debilitating illness involving a ruptured appendix and peritonitis, he was unable to tolerate the cold weather. He invariably developed chills, shivering, and muscle tension headache when exposed to the winter chill for more than several minutes. This cold sensitivity lasted for two winters following his illness after which he improved markedly. However, four years after his illness he wears much warmer clothing during the winter months than he originally required.

Symptoms and Signs

The "headache" is usually described as an aching pain in the occipital and suboccipital areas associated with a tight, pulling sensation in the posterior cervical muscles. Frequently the patient complains of a sensation of tightness involving the entire head, describing it as a "steel band" or "tight cap." Various paresthesias, such as burning of the entire scalp on combing or brushing the hair, crawling sensations, or pins and needle-like sensations may be associated. Occasionally occipital neuralgia with discomfort from the occipital nerves, commonly bilateral but occasionally unilateral, accompanies this syndrome. This is usually appreciated as a tender, aching pain following the course of the occipital nerves. The pain of occipital neuralgia may be aggravated by pressure on the occipital nerve. Procaine infiltration into the region of the occipital nerve promptly eliminates this neuralgia.

Muscle tension headache may occur at almost any time of the day or night. Most patients develop this syndrome at the end of an emotionally trying day, but we have seen this syndrome occur in the morning after a night of sleep during which the head was held in an unsuitable position for many hours. This type of headache is one of the few that is improved when the patient arises from the reclining position and sits or stands. Moving about seems to partially alleviate the pain, although at times the severe sustained contraction of the posterior cervical muscles may "fuse" the head and neck so that any movement is difficult. Sometimes this spasm extends to the masseter muscles, causing inability to open the jaws completely. Examination reveals severe muscle contraction with areas of tenderness and limitation of mobility of the head and neck. No positive neurologic changes are noted, but the deep tendon reflexes are frequently very active.

Treatment

Although muscle tension headache may be of any duration, it occasionally persists for months. To treat such a sustained headache it is advisable to hospitalize the patient.

In an attempt to promote muscle relaxation, various muscle relaxants may be used. We have found meprobamate (400 mg.) and Benadryl (50 mg.) to be effective when given four times daily. Moist heat in the form of hot towels and hot packs applied to the posterior cervical and occipital areas may aid in relaxing muscle spasm and reduce the pain. Occasionally immersion in a warm tub for one-half hour several times daily induces general muscular relaxation and alleviates the headache.

When the muscle spasm is mainly in the posterior cervical region and is associated with immobility of the cervical spine, head halter cervical traction may be helpful. Traction may also be useful if the pain is unilateral with spasm of the posterior cervical muscles on one side causing a "head tilt" to the involved side. The traction should be arranged so that the pull will be straight back without flexion or extension of the head. Depending on the size of the patient, 4 to 6 pounds of traction are used. In some cases, cervical traction increases the muscle spasm and aggravates the pain. When this occurs, increasing the traction weight by several pounds may fatigue the muscles, which may then relax. If aggravation of symptoms persists, the traction must be discontinued. Medication for muscle relaxation is always used in conjunction with traction.

When digital pressure on the scalp or posterior cervical region causes pain, the use of procaine infiltration should be considered. We find this particularly useful when the area of tenderness is well demarcated and fairly small, but we have also achieved satisfactory gains when the tenderness is rather diffuse. The technique of infiltration is fairly simple. We prefer to use fairly large volumes of a dilute anesthetic (20 to 40 cc. of a 0.5 per cent solution of procaine) in the expectation of achieving a more widespread effect than could be accomplished by lesser volumes of a more concentrated anesthetic (5 to 10 cc. of a 2 per cent solution of procaine). A fine-bore hypodermic needle is used to form the skin wheal after which a longer, larger bore needle is used to infiltrate down to the pericranium. When infiltrating the scalp, many physicians make the error of introducing all the anesthetic between the galea aponeurotica and the pericranium, which may easily be dissected apart by the anesthetic forced between these two layers. This is not harmful, and indeed some of the procaine should be introduced into this plane. However, if the entire infiltration is limited to this "false space," the painful area may not be made analgesic. Care should be taken to infiltrate the scalp itself so that the area of tenderness is subsequently numb to pinprick. In injecting the muscles in the suboccipital and posterior cervical regions, care must be taken to avoid the region of the foramen magnum and the atlas. Since the muscle spasm is almost always lateral to the midline, nothing is gained by deep infiltration of midline suboccipital muscles and the recommended procedure will avoid dangerous proximity to the foramen magnum area. It is not possible to predict with certainty the long-term effect of procaine infiltration. Some patients are benefited by one injection; others require six to eight infiltrations, which we routinely give at two-day intervals; and many are not improved. If after two infiltrations no improvement is realized, further procaine infiltration is not indicated.

We prefer not to combine procaine infiltration with massage in the belief that the anesthetized area may be overly traumatized but encourage the patients to take advantage of the pain-free interval to continue with their routine activities.

When the muscle tension headache is associated with occipital neuralgia, an occipital nerve block may be helpful both therapeutically and as an aid in diagnosis.

Occipital Nerve Block (Fig. 16). Both the greater and lesser occipital nerves are blocked. The patient should sit with the neck flexed moderately. The hair and scalp are cleansed thoroughly with a colorless antiseptic solution. The greater occipital nerve is injected just above the superior nuchal line approximately one inch from the midline (external occipital protuberance). The occipital artery can be palpated as it crosses the superior nuchal line and serves as an additional landmark, the nerve being immediately medial. A small-gauge hypodermic needle is introduced at this point, and when parasthesia along the course of the nerve is appreciated, 2 to 5 cc. of 1 per cent procaine is infiltrated. The lesser occipital nerve is also blocked immediately above the superior nuchal line and is located one inch lateral to the greater occipital nerve. A block that is performed properly will create a variable zone of anesthesia in the suboccipital and occipital areas. In cases of occipital neuralgia, occipital nerve block affords prompt relief of pain. Frequently a series of procaine infiltrations achieves relief of symptoms. These are usually given at weekly intervals, and a favorable response can be

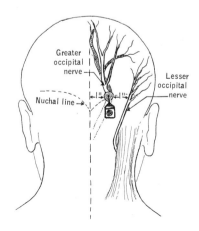

Figure 16. Technique of occipital nerve block. The greater occipital nerve is injected just above the superior nuchal line one inch from the midline. The nerve is just medial to the occipital artery, which can be palpated as it crosses the superior nuchal line. The lesser occipital nerve is blocked one inch lateral to the greater occipital nerve.

41

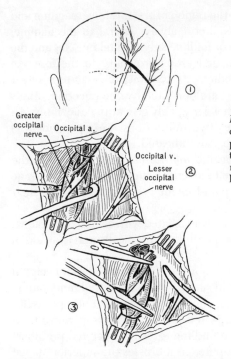

Greater
occipital
nerve
Occipital a.

Occipital v.
Lesser
occipital
nerve

①

②

③

Figure 17. Section of greater and lesser occipital nerves. (1) Incision. (2) Mass ligature placed around branches of occipital artery and the greater occipital nerve. (3) Excision of segment of neurovascular bundle and avulsion of lesser occipital nerve.

predicted by a progressively increasing duration of effect following each successive block. If after three nerve blocks the beneficial effect lasts only for the usual duration of the local anesthesia used, it must be assumed that no lasting results will be obtained. When the pain is definitely relieved temporarily by nerve block, surgical section of the occipital nerve is indicated (Fig. 17). Although this is not a difficult surgical procedure and can be performed under local anesthesia, it is best performed by a surgeon familiar with this area. One should be prepared to manage bleeding from the scalp and venous sinuses in the occipital bone.

HEADACHE DUE TO DISTURBANCES
OF THE CERVICAL SPINE

Definition

Headache can be associated with disturbances of the cervical spine in the form of acute or chronic cervical strain or arthritis of this region.

Symptoms and Signs

Such headache is invariably suboccipital and is due to irritation of the upper cervical roots, causing spasm of the posterior cervical muscles attached to the nuchal lines of the occipital bone, or to neuralgia of the occipital nerves themselves. The location of this headache is similar to that in many patients with muscle tension headache, but the two types are generally easily differentiated. The personality of the patient is not clearly neurotic, and the headache is either associated with, or preceded by, a history of cervical pain or stiff neck. The headache may follow acute cervical strain as suffered in the whiplash type of neck injury. It is aggravated by movements of the head upon the neck and these movements frequently will be limited. The head may be tilted, generally to the side of the involvement, when the pain is unilateral. X-rays of the cervical spine will show distinct arthritic changes or straightening or even reversal of the normal cervical lordotic curve. The changes noted in the x-ray will be found principally in the upper three or four cervical vertebrae, and perhaps oblique views of this area will show some encroachment upon the intervertebral foramina.

Treatment

Muscle relaxants again are helpful. The combination of meprobamate and Benadryl has been most useful in our hands. Analgesics are also helpful, and generally aspirin combined with codeine or Darvon is effective. Heat and hot packs applied to the posterior cervical and suboccipital regions may be very useful in aiding the relaxing of muscle spasm and overcoming the pain. Cervical traction should be tried in all cases. Continuous halter traction with 6 to 8 pounds for as much of the day as the patient can tolerate it is generally useful. This should be combined with periods of heavier traction as provided by the Sayre technique or some form of automatic traction by which 30 to 40 pounds of pull is applied intermittently. The traction should be arranged so that the pull will be straight along the axis of body without flexion or extension of the head. This treatment should be supplemented or followed by the use of a cervical support in the form of a collar or brace.

Specific local injections into tissues of this area are frequently helpful as described under treatment of muscle tension headache.

POST-TRAUMATIC HEADACHE
Definition

Headaches following cerebral trauma that persist long after the physical effects of the trauma (bruises, lacerations) have subsided are considered post-traumatic or postconcussion headaches.

Symptoms and Signs

Approximately 50 per cent of all patients who sustain a head injury complain of chronic, persistent headache. In our experience, these headaches have no special characteristics and exist in as many variations and combinations as the number of patients. Frequently they are associated with other

43

symptoms, such as vertigo, lightheadedness, nausea, vomiting, visual disturbances, tinnitus, impaired memory, and emotional instability.

A common misconception exists regarding a direct relationship between the extent of the injury and the severity of the postconcussion headaches. In our opinion there is absolutely no evidence that a patient who recovers from massive craniocerebral injury involving damage to the skull, dura, and cerebrum will be more likely to suffer chronic headaches than the individual who has sustained a mild concussion. At one time, it was popularly held that severe head injuries associated with blood in the spinal fluid invariably produced postconcussion headaches of prolonged duration, presumably due to adhesions between the dura and cortex resulting from the bloody spinal fluid. This theory is proved invalid if one realizes that the patient with a subarachnoid hemorrhage resulting from a ruptured cerebral aneurysm invariably is rid of his headache once the blood in the spinal fluid has been absorbed and the spinal fluid pressure has returned to normal. The patient who has undergone a craniotomy rarely complains of discomfort after the immediate postoperative interval. This evidence would argue against the theory that prolonged headaches result from damage to the brain or its protective coverings. We have noted no correlation between abnormalities in the electroencephalogram and severity of headaches.

Every physician who treats head injuries has found a suggestively high incidence of postconcussion headache in patients who have suffered an injury of an industrial or medicolegal nature, which may involve compensation. On the other side of the coin, it is rather unusual to find a patient with prolonged postconcussion symptoms resulting from an accident in the home or arising from recreational activities, which are not covered by compensation or insurance.

It should not be inferred that the majority of postconcussion headaches are based simply on the patient's desire to collect a substantial reward in return for his suffering. Among the many factors involved, the sudden accident that precipitously halts the competitive struggle of daily living creates a psychologic problem. The individual who has managed to cope adequately with the frequently stressful demands of modern civilization is given the option of honorably withdrawing from the fray, since no one could claim that the accident was of his choosing. With this consideration in mind, it is of interest to note that the passenger (not the driver), the worker who slips on the oil slick carelessly left on the floor by others—the individual who is clearly the innocent victim—is the patient most likely to suffer with chronic post-traumatic headaches. Many other latent neurotic factors, such as resentment, depression, fear, and frustration, are brought to the surface by a suitable accident. These all tend to augment the patient's symptoms, establishing a cycle resulting in prolonged, chronic suffering.

Cranial Trauma and Low Spinal Fluid Pressure Syndrome

Following a cranial trauma an occasional patient experiences an inordinate amount of headache that is particularly severe when he is in the upright position. The headache may persist for several weeks following a severe head injury that has resulted in cerebral contusions, when in other respects the patient has shown continuous improvement. It may be present shortly after what appeared to be a mild concussion and may be accompanied by nausea and blurred vision. A lumbar puncture will reveal a low cerebrospinal fluid pressure, and it can be hypothesized that the trauma has produced a local reflex vasospasm of the choroidal vessels. This would reduce spinal fluid production and result in intracranial hypotension. This syndrome is self-limited to a matter of a few days to several weeks, and in a few instances our patients with this syndrome have appeared to respond specifically to inhalations of 10 per cent carbon dioxide in oxygen.

Occipital Fractures Associated with Bloody Spinal Fluid

Severe headache persisting for several days or perhaps a week following cranial trauma in a patient who is otherwise alert should bring to mind the possibility that traumatic subarachnoid hemorrhage has occurred; evidence of meningeal irritation should strengthen this suspicion. In our experience a linear fracture of the occipital bone is most apt to be associated with subarachnoid bleeding, perhaps because of the concentration of large venous sinuses in this area. A lumbar puncture, of course, will firmly establish this diagnosis. Awareness of this diagnostic possibility in the presence of an apparently undue amount of headache following a cranial trauma has avoided concern regarding more serious diagnostic considerations or the classification of the patient as neurotic or litigation-minded.

Treatment of Post-traumatic Headaches

The use of appropriate drugs and physical methods varies according to the widely differing characteristics of the headache. If sustained muscle spasm is an associated feature, procaine infiltrations are beneficial. In some cases with migraine-like features, relief has been obtained with ergotamine tartrate. Histamine desensitization also has its place in the management of postconcussion headaches. Of prime importance in management is the complete awareness of the physician of the psychologic mechanisms contributing to the illness and his active participation to frustrate and oppose these forces. The well-meaning doctor who needlessly prolongs the period of bed rest may, by his overzealous concern, be acting against the best interests of his patient. If in 24 to 48 hours the patient's general status is such that he may be progressively mobilized, mild lightheadedness, vertigo, or pain should be no valid deterrent. A confident, cheerful attitude regarding the eventual satisfactory prognosis is of specific value in this regard.

Frequently the fuel that maintains the smoldering fire is the interminable legal mechanics involved with a compensation conflict. These issues are best settled promptly and conclusively with a termination of all courtroom and legal procedures. This is frequently difficult to accomplish, since it often runs counter to the advice of the patient's lawyer who may want to prolong the litigation in an effort to obtain a greater settlement for his client. The

45

obvious effect is to cause the patient to be consistently preoccupied with his symptoms, and this in many cases delays recovery.

HEADACHE ASSOCIATED WITH CEREBROSPINAL HYPOTENSION

Definition

There is a group of patients who complain of severe headache that is characteristically aggravated when the head is elevated, as in the upright position. In some instances the headache is only present when the patient is in the upright position.

Mechanisms

Most numerous in this category are patients with headache following lumbar puncture done either for diagnostic or anesthetic purposes. The headache that follows shortly after the procedure has been shown to result from the leakage of cerebrospinal fluid through the puncture hole in the arachnoid and dura, decreasing the intracranial pressure and leading to traction on the pain sensitive structures within the skull. However, in postspinal puncture headache that persists for more than four days, it is believed that continued leakage cannot be inferred, at least not in sufficient quantity, to explain the maintained intracranial hypotension. Rather, it must be assumed that a decreased production of cerebrospinal fluid, possibly due to a localized reflex spasm of the choroidal vessels or a disturbance of the hypothalamic centers that control spinal fluid production, supervenes upon and maintains the original hypotension that resulted from leakage of fluid. It has been amply shown that the use of a small-bore spinal needle, thereby producing a smaller rent in the dura and allowing less spinal fluid to escape, reduces the number of postpuncture headaches. When feasible, this should be used. For diagnostic purposes, however, especially to measure accurately the cerebrospinal fluid pressure and perform the Queckenstedt test, an 18-gauge needle should be used.

Treatment

It appears that the incidence of postpuncture headache is reduced by having the patient lie prone for several hours immediately after the procedure. The exact reason for this is not entirely clear but presumably the effect is related to the increased abdominal pressure, which elevates the intraspinal pressure. Once the headache appears, it is helpful to keep the patient well hydrated and to use carbon dioxide inhalations (5 per cent CO_2 in 95 per cent O_2), which the patient administers to himself by mask from a tank left at the bedside. The carbon dioxide is used at hourly intervals of five minutes' duration.

In very severe, prolonged cases, an epidural injection of 20 to 30 cc. of normal saline may produce rather dramatic relief of symptoms.

Spontaneous Intracranial Hypotension

Spontaneous intracranial hypotension characterized by headache exaggerated in the upright position, vomiting, rigidity of the neck, and some photophobia, although a relatively rare syndrome, has been widely described. Schultenbrand first hypothesized a decrease in cerebrospinal fluid production as the mechanism underlying this syndrome, but the etiology remains obscure. We have encountered six patients, all women, whose symptoms fell into this group. The use of carbon dioxide inhalations was helpful but did not appear to have permanent effect. In each instance severe headache detained the patient in the hospital two to three weeks and persisted in mild form for several weeks thereafter.

PSYCHOGENIC HEADACHE
Definition

The term *psychogenic headache* comprehends the majority of headaches complained of by patients visiting the physician. These headaches originate in the psyche or the emotional reaction of the patient and have no primary somatic origin. The classification is quite arbitrary, since several types of headaches, such as migraine, post-traumatic headache, and muscle tension headache, can be considered psychogenic.

Symptoms and Signs

Psychogenic headaches commonly start in the frontal or occipital regions and spread over the entire head. The duration and frequency of attacks may vary but tend to be extremely protracted. It is not unusual for patients to complain of a continuous headache lasting for 10 or 20 years. Although these pains vary in intensity, for the most part they are of moderate intensity and do not generally interfere with routine activities. The pain may become more severe when a break in the everyday pattern occurs, which is as likely to be a pleasurable interval as an unpleasant task. A long-awaited vacation may be delayed or postponed by a severe headache just as well as putting off a disagreeable visit to the dentist. The headache is often described as a pressure sensation; "band-like," "tingling," "uncomfortable warmth," and "pins and needles" are other terms used to describe the symptoms. When questioned closely regarding such specific items as the frequency, duration, and precise location, many patients are indefinite and reluctant to give direct answers. On the other hand, some patients furnish extremely detailed descriptions of their symptoms. One should take careful notes of the symptoms as described and compare them with the complaints offered on the next visit. A striking variation in the pattern and description of the pain is common.

47

Many patients state that aspirin or similar simple analgesics do not affect the pain. Placebo therapy may or may not be effective, but a positive response to placebos is far from conclusive evidence that the pain is psychogenic, since many patients with pain of organic etiology are relieved by this type of management.

The most important feature in diagnosing headache of psychogenic origin is a correlation of emotional disturbances and personality defects with the presenting symptoms.

Treatment

The most effective method of management of this type of headache requires a good physician-patient relationship. The patient must be made aware of the genuine interest and concern of the physician and must be confident in his proper judgment. A complete neurologic work-up, which includes skull x-rays, electroencephalography, and lumbar puncture, not only allays the patient's fear of serious organic disease but aids and strengthens the physician's clinical impression regarding the psychogenic etiology of the symptoms. In cases that are truly intractable, psychiatric care may be necessary.

chapter four

Facial Pain

chapter four —

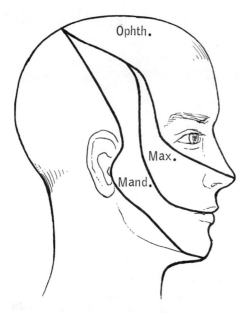

Figure 18. Sensory distribution of the trigeminal nerve.

Facial Pain

Pain affecting the face and jaw can be caused by a number of diseases and disorders all of which can be differentiated by certain distinct characteristics. The multiplicity of these disorders and the frequently confusing symptoms tax the diagnostic ability of the physician. Although medical help is now readily available, we continue to be dismayed by the numbers of individuals suffering from trigeminal neuralgia who have had needless dental extractions involving the entire upper or lower jaw and who are subjected to prolonged regimens of equally useless therapy. To avoid needless suffering, the physician must be familiar with the major causes of facial pain and the methods of treatment that provide optimal results.

TRIGEMINAL NEURALGIA

Trigeminal neuralgia or tic douloureux is characterized by recurrent, episodic attacks of extremely severe pain over the distribution of one or more branches of the fifth cranial nerve (Fig. 18). The pain occurs suddenly and without warning, usually lasts 10 to 30 seconds, and stops as abruptly as it began. Patients describe the pain as an electric shock or a shooting or jabbing sensation. The pain can occur spontaneously or may be brought on by stimulating a "trigger zone," which may exist in any part of the face. The trigger area most frequently indicates the branch of the nerve involved; otherwise it might be difficult to localize the pain precisely. The area from the lateral border of the nose to the angle of the mouth, which is supplied by the second division of the fifth cranial nerve, is the most common trigger zone (Fig. 19), but as the disease progresses, secondary trigger zones occasionally develop. The stimulus may be talking, chewing, washing the face, blowing the nose, or sometimes the lightest, almost imperceptible touch or even a draft of cool air on the face. The pain is often triggered by hot or cold food or drink. The single, momentary episode of pain may eventually

51

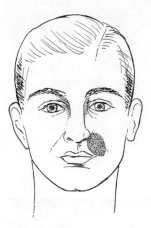

Figure 19. The most common trigger zone in trigeminal neuralgia is the area from the lateral border of the nose to the angle of the mouth, which is supplied by the second division of the fifth cranial nerve.

progress to a series of multiple single bursts, which follow one on the other for an hour or longer. After a prolonged attack of this nature, some patients complain of a mild, dull, aching pain, which may persist between attacks in the same distribution as the original short, severe pain.

The etiology of trigeminal neuralgia is unknown. Usually it occurs in patients over the age of 50 and is twice as frequent in women as in men. It is always unilateral, although in rare cases the contralateral side is affected at a later date, and most often is seen on the right side. Although the pain may disappear for several months at a time, it invariably recurs, spontaneous recovery being extremely rare. The attacks rarely awaken the patient from sleep unless the trigger zone is stimulated inadvertently.

During periods of frequent attacks, patients attempt to avoid any stimulus that may precipitate the pain. When indicating the site of pain, they avoid touching the face and attempt to speak while keeping the affected side of the face immobile. Patients frequently present themselves with a noticeable layer of grime and unshaven beard covering the involved portion of the face. When attacks are triggered by chewing or swallowing, the patient may deteriorate into an advanced state of emaciation and dehydration. In some cases the pain and suffering become intractable and, if relief is not offered, may lead to suicide.

Diagnosis

The neurologic examination is normal with intact sensation in the trigeminal area. If the pain extends beyond the anatomic distribution of the trigeminal nerve, other diseases must be considered. A variety of pathologic conditions, such as tumors, aneurysms, and toxic neuritides, may irritate the trigeminal nerve mechanically and cause dull, prolonged discomfort within the sensory field of the nerve. This is sometimes referred to as secondary trigeminal neuralgia.

Treatment

Medical Treatment. To date no drug has been developed that relieves "tic" pain for predictably sustained periods of time. The natural history of the disease with prolonged pain-free intervals has tended to create glowing reports of cures in the early stages of trial with a variety of drugs. The most that can be said for any of the drugs used is that they may effect transient and occasionally only partial relief of pain. Morphine and other analgesics are of no value because of the brief interval of the pain. When the pain occurs in prolonged paroxysms, the large amounts of morphine necessary to control pain create the danger of respiratory depression if the pain ceases spontaneously. Inhalation of trichlorethylene (15 drops several times a day) may provide remission of the pains. Large doses of thiamine chloride or vitamin B_{12} have not been effective in our hands. The most recent medication added to the list is Dilantin sodium, which is in wide use as an anticonvulsant. We have used this drug in doses of 100 mg. three or four times daily with some transient effect on several cases, but in most instances it has proved of no value.

Nerve Block. Injection of alcohol into the second and third divisions of the trigeminal nerve causes neurolysis at the site of injection, followed by degeneration of the nerve fibers peripheral to the zone of destruction. The undamaged sensory nerve cells are located above the point of injection, within the gasserian ganglion, permitting regeneration of the nerve and return of sensation (and pain) in 6 to 24 months. After the first alcohol injection the duration of relief tends to diminish with each successive injection, probably because the scar tissue resulting from the previous injection prevents proper diffusion of the alcohol. The course of the pain and location of the trigger zone indicate the proper division to be injected.

The technique of injecting alcohol into a nerve no more than 2 or 3 mm. in diameter, which is located 5 or 6 cm. beneath the surface of the skin, is difficult because the destructive properties of alcohol require accurate placement of the needle within the nerve sheath with only 1 or 2 cc. of solution used. This is in contrast to procaine injection technique, which permits the general area of the nerve to be bathed with much larger quantities of solution if a "direct hit" upon the nerve cannot be accomplished (Fig. 20). The procedure is usually performed under local anesthesia of the skin only so that the patient may report the occurrence of pain or paresthesias when

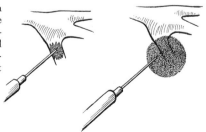

Figure 20. The technique of injecting alcohol into a nerve requires an accurate placement of the needle sheath and the use of only 1 or 2 cc. of solution. By contrast, procaine injection technique permits the general area of the nerve to be bathed with much larger quantities of solution if a "direct hit" upon the nerve cannot be accomplished.

the needle penetrates the nerve. Because injection is extremely painful and not a permanent "cure," some clinics have abandoned its use, relying on surgery exclusively. We prefer to use alcohol injection as the first stage of management for the "tic" patient who previously has not been treated definitively. We find that the annoying paresthesias associated with permanent surgical interruption of the trigeminal nerve are poorly tolerated by many patients, particularly those who are not prepared to accept this constant unpleasant sensation as a substitute for their original episodic pains. The patient who undergoes permanent trigeminal nerve interruption by surgery after the effects of an alcohol block have diminished is usually prepared to accept this side effect. Although the average case of trigeminal neuralgia is readily diagnosed and is rarely confused with other entities, an occasional atypical case is seen. If relief of pain has been afforded by previous alcohol block, surgery can be performed confidently with the knowledge that permanent interruption will produce similar relief.

First Division. As the first division of the trigeminal nerve branches out from the gasserian ganglion it courses within the cavernous sinus adjacent to the third, fourth, and sixth cranial nerves so that injection at that site is not technically feasible (Fig. 21). However, the supraorbital branch of the first division may be blocked as it curves around the supraorbital ridge or emerges through the supraorbital foramen. This nerve supplies the skin of the forehead and scalp up to the vertex. If the pain is primarily in the first division or if the trigger zone is located within the field of the supraorbital nerve, blocking this nerve may relieve the pain.

The supraorbital foramen or notch can easily be palpated 2.5 to 3 cm. from the midline. A 25-gauge hypodermic needle is inserted into the notch to a depth of 0.5 to 1 cm. (Fig. 22). Since procaine is not used, the unanesthetized nerve is contacted by the tip of the needle to produce paresthesia. The needle is firmly maintained in position while 0.5 to 1 cc. of absolute alcohol is slowly injected. This is an easily performed block without complications other than some edema of the eyelid. However, several smaller

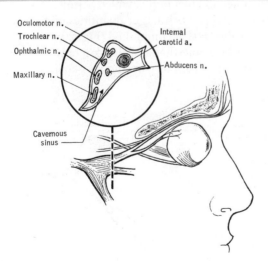

Figure 21. As the first division of the trigeminal nerve branches out from the gasserian ganglion, it courses within the cavernous sinus adjacent to the third, fourth, and sixth cranial nerves so that injection at that site is not technically feasible.

branches of the first division (infratrochlear, supratrochlear, nasal), which also curve around the supraorbital ridge as they leave the orbit, are unaffected by the block and may be a factor if the pain is not relieved (Fig. 23). Since surgical avulsion of the supraorbital nerve is a relatively minor procedure, which makes it possible to interrupt all branches, we rarely inject this branch.

Second Division. The second division of the trigeminal nerve (maxillary nerve) originates at the anterior border of the gasserian ganglion between the first and third divisions and leaves the cranial cavity via the foramen rotundum, coursing into the pterygopalatine fossa. It then passes through the inferior orbital fissure to enter the orbit where it courses along the floor of the orbit, exiting through the infraorbital foramen.

Maxillary Nerve Block in the Pterygopalatine Fossa. This block is performed with the patient in the supine position, and a sandbag is placed beneath one shoulder to facilitate lateral rotation of the head. The head rests on a firm, flat sandbag to maintain a perfect lateral position (Fig. 24). Luminal sodium (2 gr.) is administered prior to the block for sedation, since this procedure is often painful. A bite block is helpful to separate the jaws in edentulous patients, or the dentures can be worn. A three-inch, 21- or 20-gauge lumbar puncture needle is used rather than a finer needle to avoid bowing the shaft of the needle, which would hamper accurate estimation of the

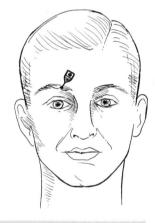

Figure 22. Technique of supraorbital block. The supraorbital foramen or notch is palpated 2.5 to 3 cm. from the midline, and a 25-gauge hypodermic needle is inserted into the notch to a depth of 0.5 to 1.0 cm. Since procaine is not used, the unanesthetized nerve is contacted by the tip of the needle to produce paresthesia. The needle is maintained in position while 0.5 to 1 cc. of absolute alcohol is injected slowly.

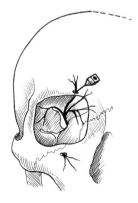

Figure 23. Position of the needle in supraorbital block.

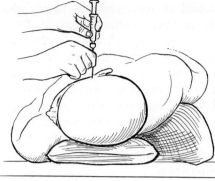

Figure 24. Proper position of the patient for maxillary nerve block in the pterygopalatine fossa or mandibular nerve block at the foramen ovale.

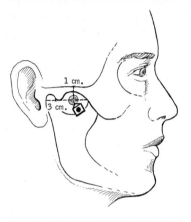

Figure 25. Maxillary nerve block. A procaine wheal is made 3 cm. anterior to the tragus of the ear and 1 cm. below the zygoma.

1 cm.

3 cm.

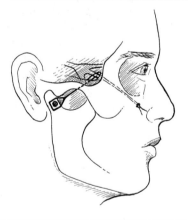

Figure 26. Maxillary nerve block in the pterygopalatine fossa.

needle tip and impair the sense of bony resistance. A procaine wheal is made 3 cm. anterior to the tragus of the ear and 1 cm. below the zygoma (Fig. 25). Prior to placing the wheal, it is helpful to mark this site with a small cross made by indenting the skin with the thumbnail. The rubber marker on the lumbar puncture needle is set at 6 cm. The needle is advanced slowly with the tip directed slightly anterior and superior so that it is pointed toward the apex of the orbit. If bone is encountered at a depth of 4 or 5 cm., the needle is impinging upon the pterygoid plate of the sphenoid bone and should be "walked" anteriorly to "fall" into the pterygopalatine fissure. Occasionally the tip may be advanced too far forward and may contact the maxilla at a depth of 4 cm. When the needle is in the pterygopalatine fossa, it should be advanced very slowly until a sudden stab of lancinating pain in the upper lip reveals the needle to be in contact with the maxillary nerve (Fig. 26). The needle is maintained completely immobile while several drops of absolute alcohol are slowly injected through the needle. A sensation of fullness and hypesthesia in the upper lip accompanied by a burning sensation as the injection is performed indicates that the needle is well placed. The third, fourth, and sixth cranial nerves are all in close proximity to the second division as they enter the superior orbital fissure so that one should be on the alert for development of diplopia or extraocular palsy as 1 cc. of alcohol is injected slowly. External rectus palsy due to involvement of the sixth cranial nerve is the most common extraocular palsy seen as a complication of this injection. This is usually transient, lasting six to twelve weeks, but if it is noted, the injection is terminated immediately.

Infraorbital Block. The infraorbital branch of the maxillary nerve can be blocked easily as it leaves the infraorbital foramen to create a small zone of numbness involving the upper lip and cheek. However, second division tic pain usually involves the palate and teeth, requiring interruption of the maxillary nerve before the alveolar nerves (anterior, middle, posterior) are given off. For this reason the more difficult pterygopalatine block is used unless the pain radiation is limited to the cheek and upper lip. Occasionally one may block the infraorbital nerve and obtain relief of pain even though the original pain involved the entire distribution of the second division. This usually occurs in patients who have a very sensitive trigger zone in the upper lip, and numbing the trigger area causes the pain to disappear. This, however, is not predictable and the duration of pain relief may vary considerably.

The infraorbital foramen is located 1 cm. below the inferior orbital rim and 2.5 to 3 cm. from the midline. It slants upward toward the orbit and slightly laterally. It is in direct line with the supraorbital notch and the pupil of the eye. A 25-gauge needle is introduced through the unanesthetized skin about 1.5 to 2 cm. beneath the inferior orbital rim and directed at a 60-degree angle toward the orbit. It is important to enter the skin slightly below the foramen to allow for the upward direction of the needle. Bone is encountered at a depth of 1 cm., and with careful probing it is a simple matter to locate the infraorbital foramen. When the tip of the needle enters the foramen, paresthesia is produced in the upper lip (Fig. 27). The needle should be advanced no farther than 0.5 cm. within the canal to avoid complications. Deeper insertion may cause the needle to penetrate the floor of the canal, which may be paper-thin or in rare instances entirely absent, leading directly into the maxillary sinus. Aspiration should be attempted prior to injecting alcohol; air drawn into the syringe indicates entrance into the sinus in which case the injection is discontinued. Rarely the needle perforates the upper wall of the foramen to enter the orbital cavity. When the needle is in proper position, 1 cc. of absolute alcohol is slowly injected.

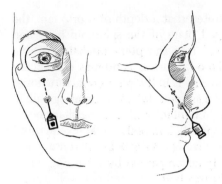

Figure 27. Block of the infraorbital branch of the maxillary nerve. The needle enters the skin slightly below the foramen to allow for the upward and lateral slant of the bony canal.

Third Division: Mandibular Nerve Block at the Foramen Ovale. The patient is prepared and positioned in the same manner as described for maxillary block in the pterygomaxillary fossa. A procaine wheal is made 2 cm. anterior to the tragus and 1 cm. below the zygoma. A 21-gauge lumbar puncture needle with the depth marker set at 5 cm. is introduced through this wheal. The needle is maintained at a right angle to the anterior-posterior plane of the face and aimed slightly cephalad so that it will almost touch the base of the skull at a depth of 4.5 to 5 cm., when it will contact the mandibular nerve after it exits from the foramen ovale. When the nerve is contacted, pain radiates to the lower lip. The needle is carefully maintained in position as 1 cc. of absolute alcohol is slowly injected (Fig. 28).

In performing this block, care must be taken to avoid penetration of the needle beyond the depth of 5 cm. to prevent injury to other cranial nerves, the cavernous sinus, and the internal carotid artery. If the needle is directed too far posteriorly, the eustachian tube may be penetrated, causing pain in the ear.

The mental nerve, a branch of the mandibular nerve, can be blocked as it exits from the mental foramen, but because of the relatively limited zone of anesthesia produced, this block is not useful in the management of trigeminal neuralgia.

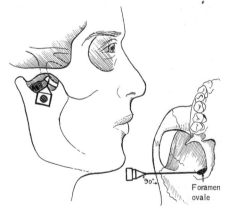

Foramen
ovale

Figure 28. Mandibular nerve block at the foramen ovale.

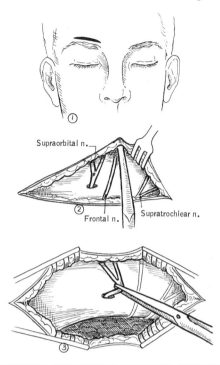

Figure 29. Supraorbital nerve avulsion. (1) The incision is made above the brow line, starting lateral to the supraorbital notch, and is carried to the medial extent of the brow. (2) A narrow periosteal elevator is used to expose the supra-orbital ridge. Care is taken to carry this exposure medially so that the frontal and supratrochlear nerves can be seen. (3) All the nerves are avulsed by twisting them about a hemostat.

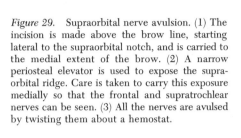

Surgery of Trigeminal Neuralgia. A variety of operative procedures can be performed for trigeminal neuralgia. Avulsion of the supraorbital and infraorbital nerves is technically simple and carries no significant risk to the patient, but with regeneration of the nerve, the pain returns. All the surgical procedures that create permanent effects are major intracranial operations and should be performed only by neurosurgeons. There is no place in medicine for the so-called courageous surgeon who performs procedures beyond his training. This sort of courage is practiced at the risk and sometimes the expense of the patient.

Supraorbital Nerve Avulsion. This is a simple procedure and is preferable to the alcohol injection, because the effective duration is longer and several additional nerve branches can be interrupted, making relief of pain more certain.

The eyebrow is not shaved, because 25 per cent of shaved brows do not regrow or regrow only partially, causing unsightly asymmetry. The incision is made above the brow line, starting lateral to the supraorbital notch, and is carried to the medial extent of the brow. The supraorbital and supra-trochlear nerves are avulsed by twisting them about a hemostat. General anesthesia is used (Fig. 29).

Infraorbital Nerve Avulsion. This procedure is performed under general anesthesia with an endotracheal tube angled away from the side of surgery (Fig. 30). The mouth is packed with gauze by the anesthetist and the gums are cleansed with aqueous Zephiran. A 3 cm. incision is made approximately 2 cm. above the gum margin in line with the supraorbital notch. The incision is carried down to the bone, and a narrow periosteal elevator is used

59

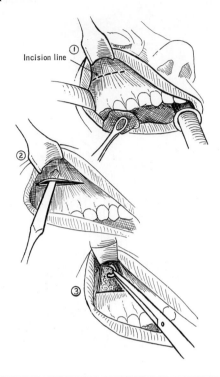

Incision line

Figure 30. Infraorbital nerve avulsion. (1) The endotracheal tube is angled away from the side of surgery. The mouth is packed with gauze. A 3 cm. incision is made approximately 2 cm. above the gum margin. (2) A narrow periosteal elevator is used to reflect the periosteum upward until the infraorbital nerve is located 1 cm. below the inferior margin of the orbit. (3) The nerve is grasped by a hemostat, which is then twisted to avulse the nerve.

to reflect the periosteum upward until the infraorbital nerve is located as it leaves the infraorbital foramen. This foramen is located 1 cm. below the inferior margin of the orbit. The nerve is grasped by a hemostat, which is then twisted to avulse the nerve. The incision is closed with a single layer of plain catgut, which is spontaneously absorbed. Normal saline mouth wash is used several times daily for three or four days postoperatively.

Retrogasserian Rhizotomy. Retrogasserian sensory rhizotomy via the temporal approach is the standard procedure used to achieve permanent relief in trigeminal neuralgia, since it is the most successful in producing permanent anesthesia and is relatively safe when performed by a trained neurosurgeon.

The operation is carried out under endotracheal anesthesia with the patient sitting in an upright position so that blood and spinal fluid will drain away to leave an unobscured operative field. Since this procedure is often performed on elderly patients who may not tolerate the sitting position while under anesthesia, we have given up the use of a dental chair, preferring an operating room table, which can be promptly adjusted to a "head down" position if the blood pressure falls precipitously. To prevent pooling of the blood in the dependent lower limbs, they are wrapped with elastic bandages prior to positioning (Fig. 31). The temporal area is shaved just prior to surgery, after questioning the patient regarding the location of pain, to avoid the possibility of operating upon the incorrect side. Proper positioning of the head is of prime importance, because any displacement, especially a lateral tilt, can easily mislead the surgeon. Once the field is draped, the operator

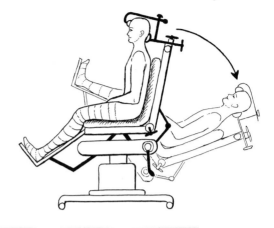

Figure 31.   Position of the patient for retro-gasserian rhizotomy. If the blood pressure falls during the procedure, the table can be adjusted promptly to a "head down" position. To prevent pooling of the blood, the dependent lower limbs are wrapped with elastic bandages.

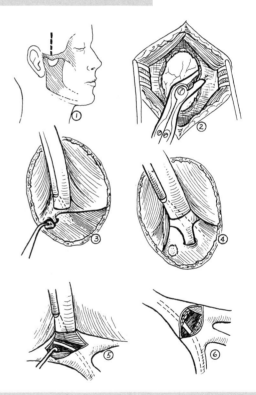

Figure 32.   Retrogasserian rhizotomy. (1) The incision is outlined 2 cm. anterior to the external auditory meatus; it starts at the lower border of the zygoma and is carried upward 8 cm. (2) A burr hole placed in the exposed temporal bone is enlarged with a rongeur. The craniectomy must be carried down to the floor of the temporal fossa for adequate exposure. (3) The dura is retracted medially, exposing the foramen spinosum through which the middle meningeal artery passes. The foramen spinosum is plugged with a wisp of cotton. (4) The foramen spinosum is identified by the small mound of packed cotton. The foramen ovale, through which the third division passes, is located 2 mm. anterior and 1 mm. medial to the foramen spinosum. (5) The dura propria has been incised, and the inferior half of the sensory roots is retracted downward and laterally, exposing the motor root, which is thicker than the sensory fibers. (6) The sensory fibers have been divided, sparing some of the ophthalmic sensory fibers in the superior and medial portions of the root sheath. The motor root is intact.

depends upon the floor and walls of the operating room to relate to the identifying landmarks so that the operating room table should not be angled but should be "squared" in the room.

The incision is outlined 2 cm. anterior to the external auditory meatus; it starts at the lower border of the zygoma and is carried upward 8 cm. It is carried no lower than the zygoma to avoid the upper branches of the facial nerve (Fig. 32). The initial incision is carried directly down to the temporal bone, splitting the temporal fascia and muscle in the direction of the fibers. A burr hole is placed in the exposed temporal bone and a craniectomy performed to the limits of the exposure. The craniectomy must be carried down to the floor of the temporal fossa for adequate exposure. The dura is carefully stripped from the squamous portion of the temporal fossa and retracted upward with a lighted retractor as the dissection is carried medially. The foramen spinosum, through which the middle meningeal artery passes, is identified and plugged with a wisp of cotton. The distal portion of the middle meningeal artery is coagulated and cut.

After cutting the artery, the foramen ovale, through which the third division passes, is located 2 mm. anterior and 1 mm. medial to the foramen spinosum. A plane of cleavage must now be developed between the dura of the temporal lobe and the epineurium surrounding the gasserian ganglion and its roots. Care must be taken at this stage to avoid traction upon the petrosal nerve, which lies posterior and lateral to the foramen ovale. This is best done by cutting the dura just anterior to the apex of the petrous bone, leaving the dura attached to the bone. Traction on this branch of the facial nerve may result in facial palsy due to secondary swelling of the facial nerve within its snug bony canal. When the ganglion and root sheath are well developed, an incision is made into the dura propria, and the tip of the lighted retractor is positioned so that it elevates the incised edge of the dura propria, exposing the sensory roots. The inferior half of the sensory root is retracted downward and laterally, exposing the motor root, which is thicker than the sensory fibers, somewhat whiter, and runs obliquely downward to reach the foramen ovale. The sensory fibers are divided, sparing some of the ophthalmic sensory fibers in the superior and medial portions of the root sheath when there has been no pain in the distribution of the ophthalmic division. Closure is performed in layers, using interrupted black silk.

When all the sensory fibers are interrupted, corneal sensation is lost. This may lead to keratitis followed by corneal scarring unless attention is given to this problem. A lateral eye shield, which can be fitted to the patient's glasses, and the use of 1 per cent methyl cellulose eye drops, which form a protective coating over the cornea, are both helpful. The most common and trying complication of trigeminal rhizotomy is continuous paresthesia in the zone of anesthesia. Sometimes this is so distressful that the patients state that they would have preferred to remain with their original tic pain. Unfortunately there is no effective treatment for this problem.

Because of these complications other surgical methods have been devised. A number of neurosurgeons are strong advocates of decompression of the gasserian ganglion or roots in which the dura is incised but the nerve fibers are allowed to remain intact. The basis for these procedures is that compression may be the etiology of tic pain. Because the recurrence rate is moderately high, we do not believe it worth the risk involved to subject the patient to a major surgical procedure, which may be a failure and necessitate a second, more difficult operation because the original tissues are distorted by scar tissue.

The descending tract of the trigeminal nerve can be cut in the medulla oblongata to produce loss of pain and temperature in the face with only slight impairment of touch. This is theoretically the most satisfactory procedure, because it eliminates the two principal complications of retrogasserian rhizotomy: corneal insensitivity and paresthesias. However, the recurrence rate is rather high, as is the operative mortality. This procedure is reserved by most neurosurgeons for the rare case in which trigeminal neuralgia reappears on the opposite side of the face after surgery on the original side has been performed. This avoids complete anesthesia of the face and the possibility of paralyzing the masticator muscles if the motor branch on the original side has been interrupted.

GENICULATE NEURALGIA

Ramsey-Hunt considered the geniculate ganglion a vestigial sensory remnant, which had been encroached upon by the trigeminal and upper cervical innervation (Fig. 33). This ever-dwindling sensory role would explain the considerable variations in the extent to which pain fibers from this ganglion innervate the deep structures of the face and head and a portion of the ear. Occurrence of severe pain in the region supplied by the geniculate ganglion is extremely rare and occurs in two forms.

Primary (Idiopathic) Geniculate Neuralgia

One form is called primary (idiopathic) geniculate neuralgia and is characterized by paroxysmal, lancinating pains within the depths of the ear. The nervus intermedius, which is the sensory portion of the seventh nerve, carries the painful impulses, which may or may not involve the anterior wall of the external auditory canal, the area just anterior to the ear, various portions of the face, as well as the deeper portion of the ear. Frequently the pain is triggered by touching certain quadrants of the external auditory canal, and cocainization of this zone may alleviate the spontaneous and induced pain for the duration of anesthesia. This condition may be confused with glosso-

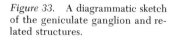
Figure 33. A diagrammatic sketch of the geniculate ganglion and related structures.

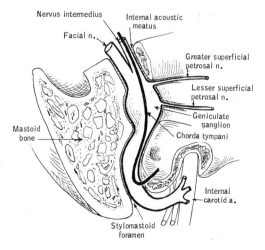

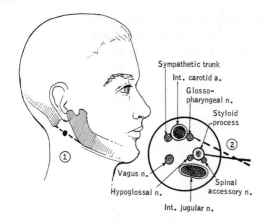

Sympathetic trunk
Int. carotid a.
Glosso-
pharyngeal n.
Styloid
process
Vagus n.
Hypoglossal n.
Spinal
accessory n.
Int. jugular n.

Figure 34. Technique of glossopharyngeal nerve block at the jugular foramen. (1) Site of the procaine wheal. (2) The needle is in contact with the styloid process. The dotted line shows the redirected course of the needle anterior to the styloid process and 0.5 cm. deeper. The proximity of the internal carotid artery and the internal jugular vein reveals the importance of testing for hemorrhage by pulling back on the barrel of the syringe prior to injecting.

pharyngeal neuralgia, which is also associated with paroxysmal pain in the ear. The differential diagnosis is made by means of glossopharyngeal nerve block at the jugular foramen (see Fig. 34), which will relieve glossopharyngeal neuralgia but not geniculate neuralgia. Intractable cases of geniculate neuralgia are treated by surgical sectioning of the nervus intermedius, although some authorities recommend cutting the glossopharyngeal nerve and the upper fibers of the vagus nerve in addition to the nervus intermedius.

Ramsey-Hunt Syndrome

Geniculate neuralgia secondary to herpes zoster of the ear is called the Ramsey-Hunt syndrome. This pain, which occurs within the depths of the ear, is usually continuous and may be very severe, often requiring large amounts of morphine. It is associated with herpetic vesicular eruptions on the tympanum and in the external auditory canal. Occasionally other portions of the facial nerve are involved with a peripheral facial palsy and loss of taste in the anterior two-thirds of the tongue. This type of geniculate neuralgia may improve spontaneously so that prior to consideration of surgery a variety of temporizing measures may be attempted. In intractable cases section of the nervus intermedius, the glossopharyngeal nerve, and the upper fibers of the vagus should be performed.

GLOSSOPHARYNGEAL NEURALGIA

Diagnosis

The pain of glossopharyngeal neuralgia occurs in burning or stabbing paroxysms much like the pain of trigeminal neuralgia. Unlike trigeminal neuralgia, the pain is appreciated in the back of the tongue, tonsillar region, posterior pharynx, and middle ear. The disease is rare, occurring one-twentieth as often as trigeminal neuralgia, and the etiology unknown. The attacks may occur spontaneously but are frequently precipitated by swallowing, talking, or touching the tonsils or posterior pharynx. A 10 per cent cocaine spray or topical application of 4 per cent cocaine may be used to anesthetize the trigger area in the back of the tongue and tonsillar area, which should cause the pains to disappear, and for the duration of anesthesia the patient may be able to swallow food and talk without precipitating the pain. Those patients who respond well to cocainization of the tonsils are treated by surgical section of the glossopharyngeal nerve intracranially.

In certain cases, when the pain is chiefly in the depths of the ear, topical anesthetization of the entire pharynx fails to relieve the pain. This might indicate that in addition to the glossopharyngeal nerve, some of the pain fibers are carried by the anterior fibers of the vagus nerve, and this is confirmed by blocking the glossopharyngeal nerve at the jugular foramen. This block affects the vagus, accessory, and hypoglossal nerves in addition to the glossopharyngeal nerve. If relief is obtained by this block, in addition to sectioning the glossopharyngeal nerve, the anterior roots of the vagus should also be cut.

Glossopharyngeal Nerve Block at the Jugular Foramen

This block is performed with the patient lying on his side (Fig. 34). A procaine wheal is made anterior to the tip of the mastoid process and just below the external auditory meatus. A 22-gauge lumbar puncture needle is introduced perpendicular to the skin until the styloid process is contacted at a depth just short of 2 cm. With the needle in this position, a marker is placed 0.5 cm. from the skin, and the needle is partially withdrawn and redirected just anterior to the styloid process until the marker is flush with the skin. Five cubic centimeters of procaine are slowly injected after first testing for hemorrhage by pulling back on the barrel of the syringe. If the vagus, accessory, and hypoglossal nerves are involved in addition to the glossopharyngeal, the patient may develop tachycardia and paralysis of the trapezius muscle and the ipsilateral half of the tongue. The cervical sympathetic chain may also be affected and cause Horner's syndrome. Because of the many structures affected by this block, alcohol is never used.

SUPERIOR LARYNGEAL (VAGUS NERVE) NEURALGIA

Diagnosis

Superior laryngeal neuralgia is extremely rare. It is characterized by severe, paroxysmal, lancinating pain in the sensory zone of the superior laryngeal nerve (base of tongue and supraglottic portion of the larynx). Wide extension of the pain may occur from the zygoma to the upper thorax. The pain may be precipitated by any activity in the throat, such as coughing, talking, swallowing, or yawning. Because of the confusing distribution of the pain, the diagnosis can be made with some degree of assurance only by blocking the superior laryngeal nerve with procaine and stopping the attack for the duration of anesthesia. The treatment is alcohol block of the superior laryngeal nerve.

65

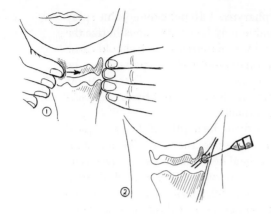

Figure 35. Alcohol block of superior laryngeal nerve. (1) The cornu of the hyoid bone is easily palpated by exerting pressure on the opposite side of the hyoid bone, causing the cornu to become more prominent. (2) The needle is inserted just inferior to the cornu and is advanced medially and slightly anteriorly.

Alcohol Block of Superior Laryngeal Nerve

The patient lies in the supine position with the head in moderate extension (Fig. 35). Do not hyperextend the neck with a sandbag beneath the shoulders, for this serves to stretch the anterolateral cervical muscles, increasing the difficulty in palpating the hyoid bone, which is used as a landmark. The cornu of the hyoid bone is easily identified by exerting pressure on the opposite side of the hyoid bone, causing the cornu to become more prominent. A procaine wheal is made just inferior to the cornu and a 25-gauge, one-inch needle is inserted through the wheal, advanced medially and slightly anteriorly. When the nerve is contacted, paresthesia radiating to the ear is elicited. If paresthesia cannot be obtained, 4 cc. of 1 per cent procaine can be injected and the solution will diffuse through the tissues. For alcohol block, however, accuracy is essential, and 1 cc. of absolute alcohol is injected only after the nerve is contacted. During the performance of the block, the patient is instructed not to swallow, speak, or cough. Because the carotid artery and jugular vein are in the vicinity, care is taken to pull back on the barrel of the syringe prior to injecting.

SPHENOPALATINE NEURALGIA

Diagnosis

Sphenopalatine ganglion neuralgia was first described by Sluder and is also known as Sluder's neuralgia. The pain is unilateral, involves the lower half of the face, and never extends above the level of the ear, giving rise to the cognomen of "lower half headache." The site of maximal pain is in the region of the orbit and the base of the nose with extension backward to the region of the ear; it is associated with a sensation of fullness in the ear and occasionally tinnitus. The pain may radiate to the neck, top of the shoulder, and rarely the entire upper extremity. The attack is frequently accompanied by rhinorrhea and nasal congestion with obstruction to nasal breathing. The duration of the attack varies from minutes to days and consists of continuous pain with episodes of lancinating pain at irregular intervals. The syndrome is twice as common in females, may be associated with menopause, and is extremely rare.

The diagnosis of this syndrome is presumably made if anesthesia of the sphenopalatine ganglion relieves the pain. Wide disagreement exists, however, on this point and also on the etiology and treatment of the syndrome. Wolff believes that the symptoms are a migraine variant due to vasodilatation of the internal maxillary artery and has reported several patients who were relieved by intramuscular injections of ergotamine tartrate. Several rhinologists are of the opinion that the disease is due to intranasal deformity and recommend submucous resection as the best method of treatment. Sphenopalatine ganglion alcohol block is the treatment favored by most and gives prolonged relief in a large percentage of cases.

Sphenopalatine Ganglion Block

This block is performed with a 1.5-inch tonsil needle. The mucous membrane medial to the last molar tooth is swabbed with aqueous Zephiran and then anesthetized topically. The tip of the angled needle is used to locate the greater palatine foramen, which is at the posterolateral angle of the hard palate just medial to the gum of the last molar tooth. The needle is then advanced along the pterygopalatine canal to a depth of 1.25 inches. Paresthesia may be elicited along the course of the maxillary nerve or the sphenopalatine ganglion. One cubic centimeter of solution is injected slowly. This injection blocks the maxillary nerve in addition to the ganglion, since both structures are adjacent to each other in the pterygopalatine fossa (Fig. 36).

Figure 36. Sphenopalatine ganglion block. (1) The needle is inserted through the greater palatine foramen. (2) Diagramatic view of sphenopalatine ganglion block.

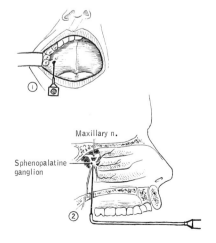

Maxillary n.

Sphenopalatine
ganglion

ATYPICAL FACIAL NEURALGIA

Persistent or remitting neuralgic pains in the face that differ from the known types of cranial nerve neuralgias have been loosely classified as atypical neuralgia. The pain of this "syndrome" is usually unilateral, deep seated, continuous, and aching. There is considerable variation in the distribution of the pain, which is rarely limited to the areas supplied by the various cranial nerves. In most cases, autonomic phenomena, such as flushing, lacrimation, conjunctival injection, congestion of the nasal mucosa, and rhinorrhea, are associated, giving rise to the prevalent opinion that the condition results from a neurovascular disorder and is related to migraine.

Diagnosis and Treatment

The diagnosis of atypical facial neuralgia is often difficult and is frequently made when the various methods of treatment for the other cranial nerve neuralgias prove ineffective. No uniform method of treatment is significantly effective, but the best results are eventually obtained with the least aggressive forms of management. With this in mind, before one considers any type of surgical attack on this problem, the patient should be exposed to extensive trials of psychotherapy and medication. Ergotamine tartrate, sedatives, muscle relaxants, tranquilizers, and antihistamines have all been successful occasionally.

TEMPOROMANDIBULAR JOINT PAIN

Signs and Symptoms

Pain produced by dysfunction of the temporomandibular joint may vary in intensity and may be intermittent or constant. It is usually described as a dull ache in the ear and lower jaw but may extend widely to involve the head, neck, and shoulder. The pain is mainly unilateral, and when the jaw is opened to the widest possible extent, the mandible is usually seen to deviate toward the painful side (Fig. 37).

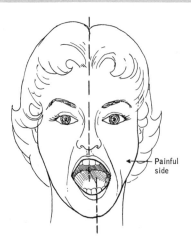

Figure 37. When the jaw is opened to the widest possible extent, the mandible usually deviates toward the painful side.

Painful side

The most frequent form of dysfunction involving the temporomandibular joint is limitation of the normal range of mandibular movement. Subluxation may also occur upon opening or closing the jaw and is marked by a sudden and involuntary jerking of the mandible or even by a sudden locking of the jaw. An instant, dull, facial pain usually accompanies subluxation and the patient may feel that the teeth no longer articulate properly.

Palpation reveals tenderness of the temporomandibular joint and the muscles of mastication (Figs. 38, 39). The patient may appreciate a click-

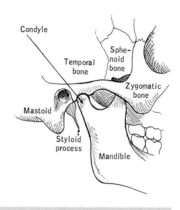

Figure 38.   The temporomandibular joint.

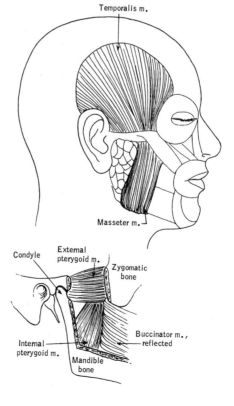

Figure 39.   Muscles of mastication.

ing in the temporomandibular joint during mastication, and the use of a stethoscope placed over the joint area during mandibular movement may reveal this sound or occasionally the sound of crepitus. When a malocclusion is present that prevents proper articulation of the front teeth, there may be an impairment in pronouncing the sibilant sounds.

Special x-ray views of the temporomandibular joint obtained with the jaw open and closed may reveal limited anterior movement of the condylar head.

Pathophysiology

The basis of most temporomandibular joint pains is usually a combination of dental malocclusion, emotional tension, and spasm of the masticatory muscles. Although the malocclusion is primarily a dental problem, this defect alone does not cause severe pain. It is generally felt that more important than the malocclusion is the emotional reaction to it and muscle spasm, which is probably secondary to emotional stress. To manage a problem of this nature the combined efforts of the dentist and the physician may be necessary.

Treatment

There is a tendency, particularly on the part of the dentist, to be overaggressive in the treatment of this problem. Many patients are markedly benefited by an understanding of the problem. To reduce emotional tension, meprobamate (400 mg. four times daily) or any of the other tranquilizers are helpful. If spasm of the muscles of mastication and other nearby muscle groups is present, Benadryl (50 mg. four times daily) can be used in conjunction with meprobamate to promote relaxation of the spastic muscles. If this combination is not successful, some of the other widely used muscle relaxants may be given a trial.

If the muscle spasm is so severe that any movement of the jaw is painful and markedly restricted, the use of local infiltration directly into the painful areas is of value. The local anesthetic used for this infiltration should be dilute (0.5 per cent procaine or 0.25 per cent lidocaine) and used in fairly large quantities (10 to 40 cc., depending upon the area involved); this is preferable to using a limited quantity of a more concentrated agent (Fig. 40).

I recall the consternation of a dentist who in the course of treating a patient for temporomandibular pain attempted to relax the spastic masseter muscle by infiltrating with the local anesthetic he used routinely for dental nerve blocks. These solutions are usually in cartridges, which fit into special syringes, are of a fairly high concentration, and are usually prepared with epinephrine. Although the patient may have had some difficulty in opening her jaw prior to the injection, following the "treatment" the reflex muscle spasm was so severe that her jaw was tightly clamped shut. As the medication was slowly absorbed, the condition corrected itself. However, such a mishap can be embarrassing and is best avoided.

Ethyl chloride spray may also be helpful in promoting relief of painful muscle spasm, particularly when the painful area is widespread and involves the cervical region and shoulder. In using this spray on the face, special precautions must be taken to avoid contact with the eyes and to prevent inhalation of the ethyl chloride fumes (Fig. 41).

Once relaxation of the muscle spasm has been achieved, the pain-free interval is utilized by moving the mandible in progressively increasing ampli-

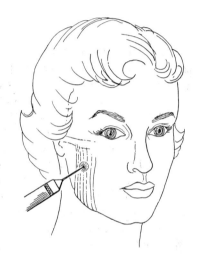

Figure 40. Infiltration of masseter and other muscles of mastication. A one inch, 25-gauge needle is inserted into the area of maximal tenderness.

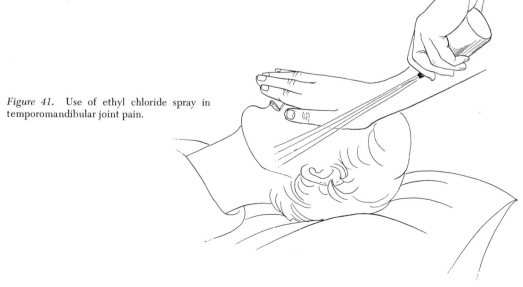

Figure 41. Use of ethyl chloride spray in temporomandibular joint pain.

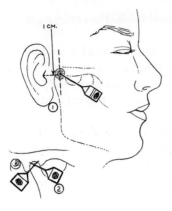

Figure 42.   Injection of the temporomandibular joint. (1) A wheal is made one fingerbreadth anterior to the tragus and just below the zygomatic arch. (2) Placement of needle behind condyle and anterior to condyle.

tudes. In initiating these exercises, the patient should gradually "warm up" the muscles before attempting to open the mouth as widely as possible. He should also attempt to open the jaw against resistance.

Occasionally arthritis of the temporomandibular joint may require injection of the joint with a local anesthetic agent. The wheal for this injection is made 1 cm. anterior to the tragus of the ear and just below the zygomatic arch. Through this wheal a 25-gauge, 2 cm. needle is introduced in a slightly posterior direction for a depth of 1.5 cm. This places the needle posterior to the condyle, and 0.5 cc. of 0.5 per cent lidocaine is injected at this site. The needle is then withdrawn into the subcutaneous tissues and redirected anteriorly so that the point is anterior to the condyle, and another 0.5 cc. of anesthetic agent is injected at this site. For severe arthritis of the joint, 10 mg. of hydrocortisone can be injected into the joint using a similar technique (Fig. 42).

Only after these measures have failed should a patient be considered for surgery of the temporomandibular joint in which the joint meniscus is excised or orthodontia is performed to correct malocclusion.

chapter five

Neck Pain and
Cervicobrachial Neuralgia

chapter five –

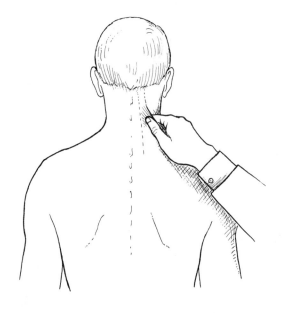

Neck Pain and
Cervicobrachial Neuralgia

The spine of man is so constructed that the ribs act as bracing struts for the thoracic vertebrae while the cervical and lumbar regions, supported only by soft tissues, are more vulnerable to stress (Fig. 43). The high incidence of pain problems occurring in the neck and low back as compared to the thoracic area demonstrates the mechanical weakness of these unbuttressed regions.

EXAMINATION OF THE NECK

A routine examination of the neck is quite easily done and if performed in an orderly fashion can be completed in five or ten minutes.

Observation

Although the patient is best examined when disrobed to the waist, adult females are apt to be self-conscious when inspected in this fashion and because of this may maintain their necks in stiff and awkward positions. To avoid this error in observation, as well as embarrassment to the patient, females are examined with their chests covered. Any deviation or straightening of the normal cervical curvature is noted (Fig. 44). The head should not be rotated or tilted to either side or inclined forward but normally rests symmetrically on the cervical spine (Fig. 45). The neck is inspected for muscle spasm posteriorly in the paraspinal muscle groups and anteriorly for prominent contracted sternocleidomastoid muscles (Fig. 46). The supraclavicular fossae are examined for abnormal prominences due to cervical

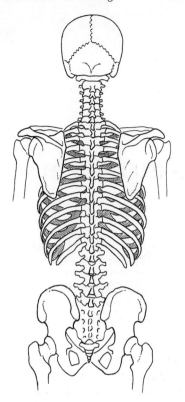

Figure 43. The ribs act as bracing struts for the thoracic vertebrae, while the cervical and lumbar regions, supported only by soft tissues, are more vulnerable to stress.

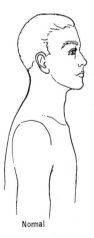
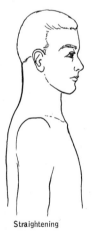

Figure 44. Straightening of the normal cervical curvature.

Normal

Straightening

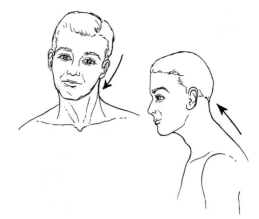

Figure 45. Head tilt and forward inclination of the head.

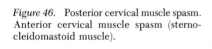

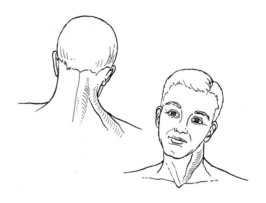

Figure 46. Posterior cervical muscle spasm. Anterior cervical muscle spasm (sternocleidomastoid muscle).

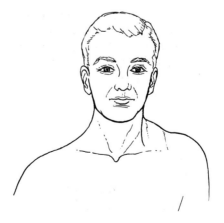

Figure 47. Shoulder elevation.

77

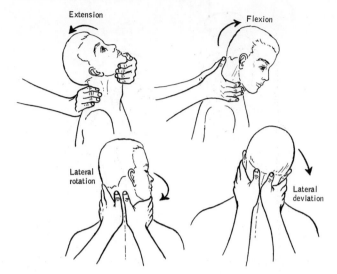

Extension

Flexion

Lateral
rotation

Lateral
deviation

Figure 48. Testing mobility of the neck.

ribs or spastic scalenus anticus muscles. The position of the shoulders is noted (Fig. 47). Is one shoulder elevated or abducted when compared with the other?

Mobility

Mobility of the neck is tested both actively by having the patient move the neck in all directions and passively by manual manipulation of the cervical spine. Extension, flexion, lateral rotation, and lateral deviation are tested. The ease and freedom of movement, pain related to specific movements, crepitation or grating during manipulation, and pain or limitation of movement on elevation of the shoulder are all noted (Fig. 48).

Palpation

Tenderness and painful muscle spasm can be determined by gentle but firm palpation. The presence of increased tissue resistance and unusually sensitive areas is noted. The posterior cervical muscles, sternomastoids, trapezii, and the scaleni in the supraclavicular fossae are palpated. The spinous process of each vertebra is palpated. When a tender, indurated nodule or area is located, it is compared carefully with the corresponding region on the opposite side.

Sensation

Keeping the sensory root dermatomes (Fig. 49) in mind, a careful sensory examination of the upper extremities is made with a pin. This is best per-

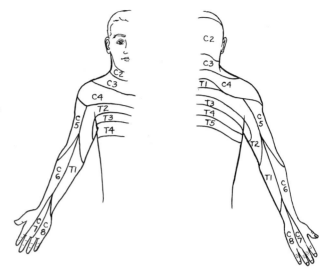

Figure 49. Cervical and upper thoracic nerve root dermatomes.

formed by examining one dermatome at a time, comparing one side with the other. In performing this examination one must attempt to maintain as consistent a degree of pressure as possible. The examiner must be aware of the principle of recruitment of stimuli by alloting an equal number of pinpricks to each side. Seven pinpricks in rapid succession will be appreciated as a stronger stimulus than five on the opposite side.

Reflexes

Deep tendon reflexes are always tested in all four extremities to establish a baseline of activity. Reflexes are tested from side to side, comparing the right

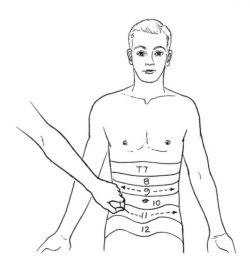

Figure 50. Abdominal reflexes are tested by scratching with a pin in the direction of the dermatome.

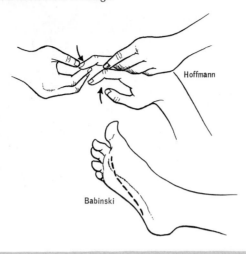

Figure 51. Hoffmann and Babinski reflexes.

biceps with the left, and so forth, rather than testing all the reflexes in one extremity before going to the opposite side.

Abdominal reflexes are tested with a pin, and the direction of the scratch is made in accordance with the sensory dermatome (Fig. 50). Test routinely for Hoffmann and Babinski reflexes (Fig. 51).

Segmental Motor Evaluation

Each major muscle and muscle grouping in the upper extremity is innervated by a "principal" or dominant nerve root. By testing the various muscles, we are able to confirm reflex and sensory findings and determine which specific nerve root is involved in lesions affecting a single nerve root. In performing these tests one side is compared with the other, and in addi-

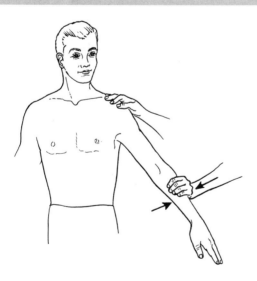

Figure 52. Testing the deltoid muscle.

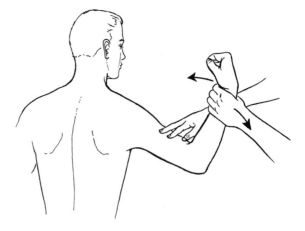

Figure 53.   Testing the biceps muscle.

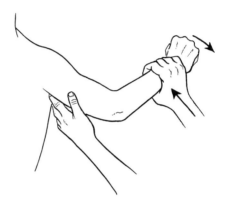

Figure 54.   Testing the triceps muscle.

tion to motor power, the examiner attempts to palpate muscle tone and mass when testing the muscle. One must remember that the root affected at the C4–C5 level is C5, that C6 is between C5–C6, and so on.

C5 (**Deltoid**).   The arm is abducted from the body, and the patient attempts to maintain that position against the examiner's resistance (Fig. 52).

C6 (**Biceps**).   The forearm is flexed at the elbow, and the patient attempts to maintain that position against the examiner's efforts to straighten the arm (Fig. 53).

C7 (**Triceps**).   The patient attempts to extend the forearm against resistance (Fig. 54).

C7–8 (**Extensors of the Wrist**).   The patient attempts to maintain extension of the wrist against resistance (Fig. 55).

C8–T1 (**Flexors of the Wrist**).   The patient attempts to maintain wrist flexion against resistance (Fig. 56).

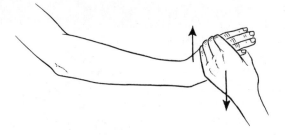

Figure 55. Testing the wrist extensors.

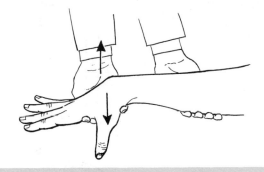

Figure 56. Testing the wrist flexors.

Radial Pulse Changes with Postural Maneuvers

The radial pulse is palpated and compared bilaterally, first with the upper extremities in a dependent position and then elevated above the head.

CHRONIC CERVICAL MUSCLE SPASM

The type of neck pain most frequently encountered is that due to chronic spasm of the posterior cervical muscles. People in occupations requiring prolonged periods of postural strain upon the neck muscles, such as draftsmen, typists, and clerks, are particularly prone to this syndrome. Equal in importance to mechanical considerations, such as posture, are emotional stress and tension. Severe cold, fatigue, and chronic eye strain are other contributory factors.

Symptoms and Signs

The patient complains of aching pain associated with a sensation of tightness in the posterior cervical region. Because the muscle spasm is sometimes extensive, discomfort may be appreciated in the occipital and suboccipital regions of the skull as well as in the trapezii and other shoulder muscles. The mobility of the neck is almost always limited to some extent, and in certain severe cases the limited mobility actually extends to the head and jaw. Palpation invariably reveals tenderness, which may be diffuse or limited to a single "trigger spot."

Fibrositis. Patients with long-standing, chronic muscle spasm frequently manifest tender areas that feel thickened, and occasionally actual nodules can be palpated within the tender muscles. The diagnosis of fibrositis can be used in these cases regardless of the objections of those who refuse to consider this a proper disease entity. The principal objection to the use of this term is the lack of pathologic proof, since histologic studies show no evidence of muscle degeneration or inflammation. There seems little question, however, that such a distinct clinical syndrome does exist, affecting the posterior cervical musculature as well as other muscles of the body. The symptoms are mainly pain, stiffness, and tenderness. The chief characteristic that distinguishes this entity is the aggravation of symptoms by inactivity and improvement with movement. A patient with fibrositis involving the posterior cervical musculature whose symptoms appear in the course of work requiring a prolonged period of concentration over a desk or drawing board or upon arising after a night's sleep will be in considerable discomfort for a while. After moving about, the stiffness subsides and the discomfort lessens. The presence of fibrositis in chronic cervical muscle spasm is usually an indication that the forms of therapy which are helpful for the milder varieties of chronic cervical muscle spasm will not be adequate. It will be necessary to employ those measures recommended for the moderate and severe grades of muscle spasm.

Treatment

The management of this disease varies according to the severity of the symptoms.

Mild Symptoms. Many patients with mild symptoms respond well to muscle relaxants and assurance by the physician, after a careful examination, that they are merely suffering from muscle spasm. It must be kept in mind that the personality of the patient and environmental tension play a considerable role in producing this symptom. A careful explanation of the psychic factors producing the disease is frequently of benefit in allaying fears regarding prognosis and may be instrumental in modifying the patient's activities to lessen emotional stress. In this connection, if the various muscle relaxants are not of benefit, a combination of meprobamate (400 mg. three times daily) and Benadryl (50 mg. three times daily) may be useful for muscle relaxation as well as tranquilization.

Moderate Symptoms. *Heat.* Heat is the most common physiotherapeutic measure applied to muscles in spasm, and the patient with posterior cervical spasm of some severity almost instinctively applies heat, using hot towels, heating pads and lamps, or exposure to sun. There is no advantage to any specific type of ordinary heat production, and the advocates of moist heat as opposed to dry heat or vice versa do not support their choice in controlled experiment. Certain forms of diathermy, however, supply deep heat to muscles through greater penetration and may be superior to ordinary heat.

In general, any form of heat that reaches the right spot may provide fairly prompt relief of pain and stiffness. The heat should be gentle and never so intense that the skin is injured. Although the application of heat may provide fairly rapid relief of symptoms, when the heat is discontinued the patient is likely to appreciate his original discomfort almost as promptly. However, regular intervals of temporary relief may act in a reflex fashion to break up the cyclic phenomenon that perpetuates the spasm. If the symptoms are improved with heat, this measure should be employed several times daily.

Ethyl Chloride Spray. When the area of tenderness and muscle spasm is localized or when a "trigger point" is present, the use of ethyl chloride spray to produce local refrigeration may be helpful. The dispenser is held upside down about 12 inches from the area to be refrigerated and moved slowly back and forth across the involved area. The refrigeration should not be continued long enough to injure the skin or underlying tissues; 15 or 20 passes are usually adequate. The patient should move his head gently back and forth as the spray is administered. When using this agent, the physician must keep in mind the general anesthetic properties of the gas. A well-ventilated room, avoidance of use of the spray in the vicinity of the nose and mouth, and protection to the eyes, which would be irritated by the spray, are routine precautions. Although the gas is not explosive, it is flammable, and therefore neither the patient nor the physician should smoke during the treatment.

Relief of symptoms, if obtained by this measure, may last from less than an hour to days. If the pain returns, the refrigeration is repeated with the hope that the pain-free intervals will progressively increase in duration. If no improvement is realized or if on repeated treatments the relief remains of brief duration, it is not likely that this method will be effective.

The local refrigeration is presumed to suppress activity of the noxious impulses that stimulate the reflex causing the spasm of the posterior cervical muscles. However, since the benefits of ethyl chloride spray vary widely in each case, there is no way of predicting in advance which patient may be relieved by this method.

Severe Symptoms. *Infiltration of Local Anesthetics.* Occasionally long-standing, chronic cases of posterior cervical muscle spasm are so severe that all the methods used to treat the milder forms of this disease are of little help. Infiltration of procaine or xylocaine into the painful areas is frequently followed by prompt relief of symptoms, which can be of prolonged duration. The presumed effect of this method is suppression of spasm-stimulating impulses from so-called trigger zones. When the pain returns, the injection is repeated, and if successful, the intervals between injections will be progressively greater.

Since the medication tends to act as an irritant, which may cause increased muscle spasm before its effect sets in, it is advisable not to use concentrations of anesthetic greater than 0.5 per cent procaine or 0.25 per cent lidocaine to avoid the possibility of causing even more severe symptoms than originally found. Epinephrine should not be added to the local anesthetic used for infiltration of spastic muscles, because the local vasoconstriction caused by epinephrine tends to prevent rapid diffusion of the anesthetic and is an undesired effect. The needle should be relatively thin (22-gauge) to avoid unnecessary trauma to the muscle. The midline is avoided to prevent damage to the cord; prior to infiltrating, the barrel of the syringe is withdrawn to avoid injection into a vessel (Fig. 57).

   Massage.   Massage of the posterior cervical muscles is usually of benefit in relieving symptoms. In addition to causing a diminution of spasm of the underlying muscles, subcutaneous adhesions resulting from chronic muscle spasm may be stretched. The muscle in spasm is manipulated firmly but gently with a kneading motion of the fingers of both hands. Although such manipulation of spastic muscles can be exquisitely painful, the kneading should not be so vigorous that it causes discomfort to normal nonspastic muscles. If this treatment is administered in too forceful a manner, the effect may be to increase the muscle spasm, worsening an already uncomfortable situation. I have occasionally found it useful to pull up a generous fold of skin and subcutaneous tissue and "roll" this fold over the painful site (Fig. 58). This particular maneuver may be extremely painful if subcutaneous

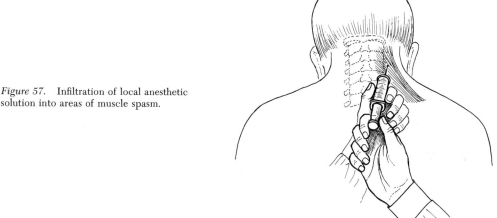

Figure 57.   Infiltration of local anesthetic solution into areas of muscle spasm.

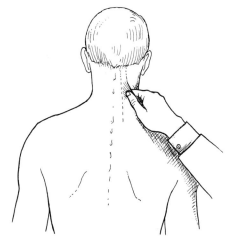

Figure 58.   "Rolling" a fold over area of muscle spasm and myositis.

85

adhesions are present, but repeated attempts become successively less uncomfortable. Muscle massage is combined with gentle manipulation of the neck in all directions.

ACUTE CERVICAL STRAIN

Any abrupt, forceful movement of the neck that occurs before a reflex protective fixation of the cervical musculature has had time to become established is capable of causing acute cervical strain. At one or another time, almost everyone has had a minor episode of this syndrome produced by an involuntary, sudden turn of the head in response to an unexpected stimulus, such as a startling noise. A sudden spasm of the posterior cervical muscles, which is invariably unilateral, results. Discomfort is appreciated in the area of spasm and a rotation or tilt of the head is seen. The symptoms of such a relatively minor episode are generally limited in duration to less than a day, after which the patient is free from symptoms.

Trauma is by far the most common cause of acute cervical strain. The trauma may consist of a blow to the head, which causes sudden hyperpositioning of the cervical spine. Loss of balance may cause a sudden twisting movement of the neck as part of the labyrinthine righting reaction in a reflex effort to regain equilibrium. This postural reaction, which is particularly well developed in cats, utilizes the neck proprioceptors as well as the semicircular canals, eyes, and medullary-spinal righting centers. Such an involuntary reflex movement of the neck occurs before the cervical muscles have had time to establish a protective fixation, causing the cervical ligaments and muscles to be strained.

Severe bodily impacts causing a snapping or whiplash movement of the cervical spine are also frequent causes of acute cervical strain. This impact may occur from a fall in which the sudden deceleration resulting from striking the ground produces hypermobility of the neck. A large number of acute cervical strains occur when the car occupied by the patient is struck forcibly from behind or on the side by a second vehicle. This type of mishap frequently occurs when the first vehicle is stopped for a traffic light and the occupant is completely relaxed and unprepared for the ensuing accident caused when the driver of the second vehicle neglects to stop in time. The lack of protective fixation of the cervical musculature at the time of the accident seems to play as great a role in the development of symptoms as the force of the blow itself. The long, drawn out legal proceedings attendant on this type of accident have projected the syndrome into a conspicuous place in the minds of physicians and lawyers. The term "whiplash" has assumed a sort of household utility since it was first introduced in an article published in the J.A.M.A. in 1953, entitled "Common Whiplash Injuries of the Neck," by Gay and Abbott.

Pathophysiology

The large variety and varying severity of mishaps that can produce acute cervical strain may cause symptoms ranging from mild to severe. The popular conception of the head's "snapping back" to a position of hyperextension is not completely correct. Study of "slow motion" films reveals that frequently a position of acute flexion occurs when a car is struck forcefully by another vehicle from behind or from the side. This is followed rapidly by extension of the head, and several oscillations of the head, back and forth, may occur, depending on the force of the original impact. The effect of this rapid, passive or nonvoluntary hypermobility of the cervical spine is to stretch the muscles and ligaments of the neck. The posterior cervical muscles are most frequently involved, and if the anatomy of these is reviewed, it will be noted that they extend from the occipital or suboccipital portion of the skull to the upper thoracic region or the shoulder girdle. The chief function of all the muscles that are closely applied to the laminae and spinous processes of the cervical vertebrae is to extend the cervical spine and head. This is the reason for the old term, "erector spinae," which is still used to refer to the superficial portion of the paraspinal muscles.

Cervical Musculature (Fig. 59)

I. Superficial Lateral
   Splenius capitis
      Origin. Lower half of ligamentum nuchae; spines of seventh cervical and first three dorsal vertebrae.
      Insertion. Mastoid process and outer third of middle oblique line of occiput.
   Splenius cervicis
      Origin. Spinous processes of third to sixth dorsal vertebrae.
      Insertion. Transverse processes of upper three or four cervical vertebrae.
   Iliocostalis cervicis
      Origin. Angle of middle and upper ribs.
      Insertion. Transverse processes of middle cervical vertebrae.
   Longissimus cervicis
      Origin. Transverse processes of upper thoracic vertebrae.
      Insertion. Transverse processes of upper and middle cervical vertebrae.
   Longissimus capitis
      Origin. Transverse processes of upper thoracic and transverse and articular processes of lower and middle cervical vertebrae.
      Insertion. Mastoid process.
II. Deep Lateral. The cervical intertransversarii muscles are vertical bands that pass between transverse processes of contiguous vertebrae.
III. Superficial Medial
   Spinalis cervicis
      Origin. Spinous processes of fifth, sixth, and seventh cervical and first two dorsal vertebrae.
      Insertion. Spinous process of axis and sometimes of third and fourth cervical vertebrae.
IV. Deep Medial
   Semispinalis capitis
      Origin. Transverse processes of five or six upper thoracic and four lower cervical vertebrae.

87

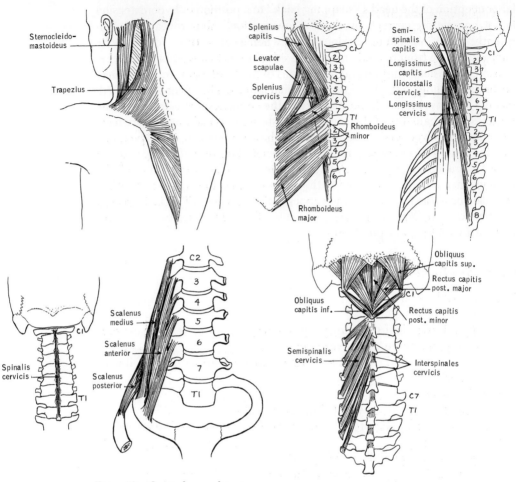

Figure 59. Cervical musculature.

Insertion. Occipital bone between superior and inferior curved lines.

Semispinalis cervicis

Origin. Transverse processes of four upper dorsal and articular processes of four lower cervical vertebrae.

Insertion. Spinous processes of second to fifth cervical vertebrae.

Interspinales cervicis. Consist of short fasciculi that extend from the upper surface of the spine of each vertebra near its tip to the lower surface of the spine of the vertebra above.

V. Suboccipital Muscles

Rectus capitis posterior major

Origin. Spinous process of axis.

Insertion. Below inferior curved line of occipital bone.

Rectus capitis posterior minor

Origin. Tubercle on dorsal arch of atlas.

Insertion. Below inferior curved line of occipital bone.

Obliquus capitis inferior
   Origin. Spinous process of axis.
   Insertion. Transverse process of atlas.
Obliquus capitis superior
   Origin. Transverse process of atlas.
   Insertion. Occipital bone below superior curved line.
VI. External Cervical Fascia and Shoulder Girdle Musculature
Sternocleidomastoideus
   Origin. Two heads, sternum and clavicle.
   Insertion. Mastoid process and outer portion of superior oblique line of
      occipital bone.
Trapezius
   Origin. Superior curved line of occipital bone, ligamentum nuchae,
      spinous processes of last cervical and all thoracic vertebrae.
   Insertion. Clavicle, spine of scapula, and acromion.
VII. Scalene Musculature
Scalenus anterior
   Origin. Upper surface and inner edge of first rib.
   Insertion. Transverse processes of third to sixth cervical vertebrae.
Scalenus medius
   Origin. Upper surface of first rib.
   Insertion. Transverse processes of second to sixth cervical vertebrae.
Scalenus posterior
   Origin. Outer surface of second rib.
   Insertion. Transverse processes of two or three lower cervical vertebrae.
VIII. Deep Musculature of the Shoulder Girdle
Rhomboideus minor
   Origin. Spines of seventh cervical and first thoracic vertebrae.
   Insertion. Scapula.
Rhomboideus major
   Origin. Spinous processes of first five thoracic vertebrae.
   Insertion. Inner border of scapula below spine.
Levator scapulae
   Origin. Transverse processes of four upper cervical vertebrae.
   Insertion. Posterior edge of scapula.

The rather wide extent of the musculature involved in supporting the cervical spine gives rise to discomfort over a large area (Fig. 60). Only the mild form of acute cervical strain produces symptoms limited to the posterior cervical region. It is much more common for the pain to extend from the occipital area down to the midthoracic region and laterally to both shoulders. The intensity of pain in the different muscle groups varies according to the specific type of accident.

The occipital and suboccipital region, with many muscles attaching, is a common site of discomfort. The wide degree of mobility in the occipital area that exists under normal circumstances tends to add impetus or augment hyperpositioning during an accident, resulting in an acute muscle stretch.

In addition to the discomfort produced by overstretched muscles and

89

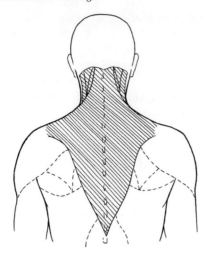

Figure 60. The wide extent of the musculature involved in supporting the cervical spine gives rise to discomfort over a large area in conditions causing muscle spasm.

ligaments, a sharp pain extending from the occipital to the parietal region is sometimes appreciated. This pain in the distribution of the occipital nerve is an occipital neuralgia secondary to spasm and edema of the suboccipital muscles, creating pressure upon this nerve.

Pain extending down one or both upper extremities may occur, particularly when the acute cervical strain is severe. This radiating pain may or may not be associated with sensory phenomena, such as numbness and paresthesias, or the sensory symptoms may be predominant with little or no actual pain. Two distinct mechanisms can give rise to pain of this nature. Spasm and edema of the scalene muscles, particularly the scalenus anticus, may cause pressure upon the brachial plexus. This problem is more likely to arise if the so-called "shoulder outlet," or the passageway through which the brachial plexus and the subclavian vessels enter the arm, is partially constricted. This constriction can be in the form of an anatomic variant, such as a cervical rib or an unusually long transverse process arising from the seventh cervical vertebra. A fibrous band extending from the tip of the seventh cervical transverse process to the first rib, or even a somewhat thickened and hypertrophied scalenus muscle, can also act as a constrictive force. Under normal conditions this limited area may be adequate to permit the brachial plexus to pass without undue pressure, but when further impingement is caused by spasm and edema of the scalenus anticus muscle, the brachial plexus is compressed.

Radiation of pain into the upper extremity may also be produced by trauma to one or more cervical nerve roots. These structures pass out of the spine through intervertebral foramina, which are formed by two adjacent vertebrae. It is conceivable that an acute angulation of the bony spine may cause impingement upon the nerve root as it passes between two affected vertebrae. A more likely cause of nerve root compression is synovitis of the interlaminar joints secondary to the trauma of severe hyperpositioning of the cervical spine. This is associated with synovial swelling, which would compress the nerve root within the intervertebral foramen. Herniation of

90

a cervical disc could result from an accident producing an acute cervical strain and would cause nerve root pressure similar in every respect to synovial swelling.

Lightheadedness, unsteadiness, and occasionally true vertigo occur to a variable degree in most individuals with acute cervical strain. This is usually due to immobilization of the neck by the spastic cervical musculature. This rigid state prevents the discrete, imperceptible, reflex neck movements that are important in maintaining body equilibrium in conjunction with the cerebellum, the inner ear, and the eyes.

Symptoms and Signs

The most striking and characteristic feature of acute cervical strain is the progressive worsening of symptoms. Immediately after the accident it is common for the patient to lightly dismiss or even completely ignore any disability relating to the cervical spine. Such statements as "My neck seemed a little stiff at the time but I thought nothing of it" or "In the excitement of the accident I did not think I was hurt" are frequently elicited in the history 48 to 72 hours later, when symptoms are quite severe. This sequence of events is thought by some physicians to prove the dishonest exaggeration of complaints by individuals who, after thinking the matter over would use the accident as a lever for personal gain. The medicolegal phase of the "whiplash injury" has been extensively discussed in many articles, most reporting that a large percentage of individuals who had prolonged symptoms were significantly relieved following settlement of litigation.

I have seen many individuals who were brought into the receiving ward following an accident because of a variety of injuries unrelated to the cervical spine. The primary trauma that occasioned admission to the hospital may clear completely within a day or two, and the patient may continue to manifest symptoms of acute cervical strain. If personal gain were the prime cause of the persistence of symptoms, the patient would likely cling to complaints related to the more obvious admitting symptom rather than elect a pain arising from a distant area.

The symptoms of acute cervical strain may be divided into three phases.

Acute Phase. Immediately after the accident the patient is usually confused and bewildered. He may note a mild discomfort in the posterior cervical region, which is described as a pulling sensation or a slight stiffness of the neck. Depending upon the severity of the trauma and the associated injuries, the duration of the acute phase varies from several hours to one or two days.

Post-traumatic Phase. This phase is marked by spasm of the cervical musculature. Moderate to severe aching pain occurs mainly in the posterior cervical region. Mobility of the cervical spine is impaired. Occipital and sub-occipital headache is usually present to some degree, and this may be associated with occipital neuralgia. The pain may radiate down one or both upper extremities if the trauma is particularly severe. Examination may reveal tenderness and spasm of the cervical musculature with fixation of the head and neck.

91

Chronic Phase. Symptoms persisting beyond two or three weeks can usually be considered to fall within the chronic phase of acute cervical strain. The posterior cervical pain from muscle spasm has usually lessened but because of its persistence may be quite annoying. With improvement in the neck pain the occipital and suboccipital discomfort may assume a major role and the patient may consider headache the predominant symptom. It is during this phase that the patient may first be aware of impairment of equilibrium with vertigo and lightheadedness. Vertigo probably occurs at this late phase only because the patients tend to limit their movements within the first week or two, and as they increase their activities they develop lightheadedness. If they do not limit activities at onset of symptoms, vertigo is likely to be appreciated initially. Nervous symptoms, such as emotional instability, insomnia, and excessive perspiration, are apt to be reported at this phase.

Management

The care of a patient with an acute cervical strain should begin as soon as possible after the accident. It is possible that by recognizing the picture in the acute phase, before the symptoms have fully developed, and initiating treatment promptly, the extent of discomfort will be reduced appreciably. When the symptoms are minimal, the patient is instructed to remain at bed rest at home. Local heat applied to the back of the neck and shoulders is helpful, and this is best administered by means of a heating pad or heat lamp. Muscle relaxants are prescribed in fairly heavy dosage and are continued in spite of temporary relief of symptoms. For pain, the patient may be given aspirin with or without codeine. Bed rest may be discontinued 24 hours after relief of symptoms. The medication is continued on an ambulatory basis and withdrawn if the patient remains symptom-free for another 24 hours.

Hospitalization is recommended for management of severe acute cervical strain. The initial care is similar to that recommended for mild cases in addition to the use of cervical traction. There are several varieties of cervical traction sets that can be adjusted to a non-hospital bed for utilization in the home. If hospitalization is not desired, this apparatus can be given a trial in the patient's bedroom. Many patients are less than faithful when treated with cervical traction at home and tend to release themselves from the chafing and annoying head halter to answer the phone and door bell, visit the bathroom, go to meals, get up for between meal snacks, and for many other excuses too numerous to mention. Because my experience with the use of home traction is generally unsatisfactory, I prefer to hospitalize any patient who is uncomfortable enough to require this form of treatment.

Every patient hospitalized with acute cervical strain should have x-rays of the cervical spine including special views for cervical ribs.

For optimal results in using cervical traction, a few simple rules should be kept in mind (Fig. 61).

1. Weight. Six to 8 lb. is usually adequate.
2. Position of the head. The head should be in a "neutral" position without flexion or extension during traction.

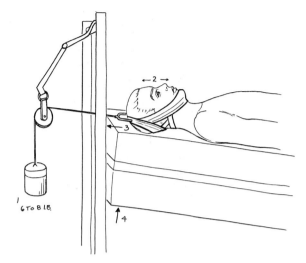

Figure 61. Halter cervical traction. (Numbers refer to explanations in text.)

3. Direction of "pull." The plane of traction force should be level with the mastoid processes. The direction of the traction should be straight back in a horizontal line from the mastoid process.

4. Countertraction. The patient tends to be pulled toward the direction of traction if the bed is level. A slight elevation of the head of the bed neutralizes this tendency; the weight of the patient's body furnishes countertraction.

5. Duration of traction. The patient is allowed to remove the traction for meals and is not required to sleep in traction.

Physical Measures for Control of Muscle Spasm. Heat and gentle massage used concomitantly are generally effective. As with chronic cervical strain, relief of pain following heat and massage is of short duration, but if any significant improvement is obtained by these means, this treatment should be continued at least twice daily.

Local Anesthesia. The use of ethyl chloride spray is not generally effective because in most cases the zone of discomfort is too widespread to be treated in this fashion. If, however, a limited area of pain and tenderness is present, this form of cutaneous anesthesia can be given a trial.

Local Infiltration of Anesthetic Agents. The use of 0.5 per cent procaine or 0.25 per cent xylocaine is frequently of great benefit in the treatment of acute cervical strain. This is best used in conjunction with massage and gentle passive and active movement of the neck. The infiltration is best accomplished with the patient prone. A pillow beneath the chest allows the patient to assume a comfortable position of moderate cervical flexion.

Suboccipital Headache. Procaine infiltration into the muscles and tendons attaching to the occiput is generally effective in diminishing discomfort in this region. The landmarks of the occipital bone must be held in mind to avoid placing a needle within the foramen magnum and causing damage to the medulla oblongata, which could prove fatal. The external occipital protuberance is only 4 cm. distant from the posterior rim of the foramen magnum. Since most of the muscles attach at the superior nuchal line, there is no need to skirt this dangerous zone.

93

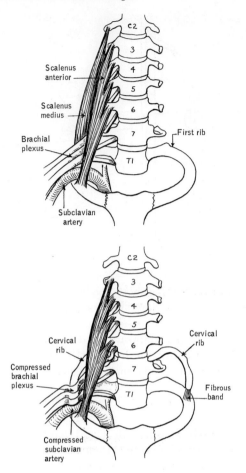

Figure 62. The "shoulder outlet" region. A spastic scalenus anterior muscle or a cervical rib can clearly cause compression of the brachial plexus and subclavian artery.

Occipital Neuralgia. Occipital neuralgia is frequently associated with suboccipital headache. An occipital nerve block should be performed as part of the local infiltration of the occipital musculature.

Pain Radiating Into the Upper Extremities. This pain can be caused by pressure upon the brachial plexus secondary to an inadequate "shoulder outlet" caused by spasm of the scalenus anticus muscle, or a nerve root may be compressed as it exits through the intervertebral canal. Of course, a careful differential diagnosis between these two separate mechanisms must be made before considering therapy.

Shoulder Outlet Insufficiency Syndrome. This syndrome is more likely to occur if the region through which the brachial plexus and vessels pass is somewhat constricted by an anatomic variant, such as a cervical rib, an elongated seventh cervical transverse process, or a fibrous band extending from the tip of the seventh cervical transverse process to the first rib (Fig. 62). Under normal circumstances this limited passageway may be adequate for the nerves and vessels to pass into the arm, but spasm and edema of the scalene muscle may augment the stricture to cause the following symptoms of pressure upon the brachial plexus:

Pain. Pain in the shoulder and supraclavicular region is dull and aching. The radiating pain may be described as boring, burning, or sharp and lancinating and usually extends down the ulnar side of the arm and hand. The pain is not aggravated by sneezing, coughing, or straining at stool.

Paresthesia. Numbness and tingling are usually present along the ulnar side of the hand, including the fourth and fifth fingers. This paresthesia, however, may involve the radial side of the hand and, in some cases, there is involvement of both sides, which is frequently described as a sensation of heaviness of the entire extremity (Fig. 63).

Sensation. Sensory examination of the involved extremity by pinprick may reveal minimal changes; frequently no sensory changes can be demonstrated.

Tenderness. Palpation of the supraclavicular fossa reveals tenderness over the scalenus anticus muscle, which, when compared with the unaffected side, gives a sensation of fullness or abnormal prominence (Fig. 64). This muscle is palpated by placing the thumb one fingerbreadth above the clavicle and forcing the posterior border of the sternocleidomastoid muscle medially.

Vascular Changes. Vascular changes are noted. Changes in the skin temperature and the radial pulse on the affected side are compared with those of the opposite side.

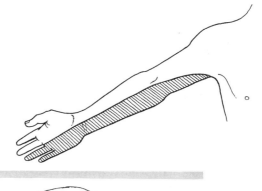

Figure 63. The numbness and tingling associated with the scalenus anticus syndrome are usually present along the ulnar aspect of the arm, forearm, and hand.

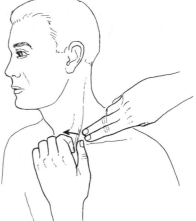

Figure 64. Palpation of the scalenus anterior muscle.

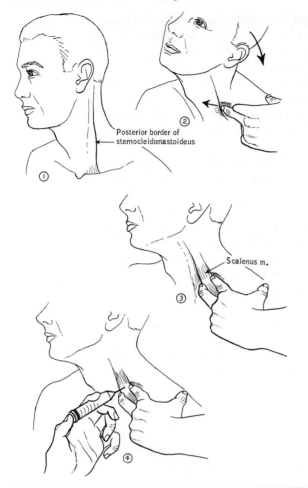

Posterior border of
sternocleidomastoideus

Scalenus m.

Figure 65. Technique of infiltrating spastic scalenus anterior muscle. (Numbers refer to steps outlined in text.)

Infiltration of the Scalenus Anticus Muscle. If spasm of the scalenus muscle appears to be the cause of pain radiating down the upper extremity, a diagnostic block of this muscle is carried out (Fig. 65). The technique of the block is designed to avoid contacting the brachial plexus or the cervical sympathetic chain with local anesthesia. If these structures are involved in the block, relief of pain may occur and the physician will have the false impression that relaxation of a contracted scalene muscle has given relief of symptoms, whereas the pain relief was actually due to sympathetic or brachial plexus anesthesia. For this reason, relief of pain following this block, if accompanied by Horner's syndrome or by anesthesia in the arm and hand, is disregarded from a diagnostic viewpoint and the block must be repeated on another occasion.

As shown in Fig. 65 (1), the posterior border of the sternocleidomastoid muscle is identified as it inserts at the clavicle. (2) The middle finger is used to push this edge of the muscle anteromedially while the patient's head is tilted toward the involved side to relax the sternocleidomastoid muscle. The patient is told to breathe in and out deeply to identify the scalene muscle, which tightens with each inspiration. (3) The scalene muscle is then straddled by the middle and index fingers as the head is tilted away from the involved side. Exerting firm pressure on either side of the scalenus anticus muscle causes the muscle belly to bulge forward. (4) A one-inch needle is inserted directly into the muscle and 5 cc. of 0.5 per cent procaine or xylocaine is injected. The short needle and limited amount of anesthetic agent are particularly important when performing the initial or diagnostic block.

Relief of radiating pain should occur within five minutes after a properly performed block if the diagnosis of scalenus anticus spasm is correct. In many cases the single block is sufficient to relax the reflex scalene spasm, achieving permanent relief of pain. If the pain does recur, several additional blocks may be necessary. Once the diagnosis has been established, 10 cc. of 0.5 per cent procaine or xylocaine may be used for subsequent blocks with the hope that more profound muscle relaxation of longer duration may be achieved.

Patients occasionally develop a severe scalenus anticus syndrome in association with acute cervical strain, which continues to recur after the effects of the local anesthetic subside. It is well to persist with local blocks, especially if progressively increasing periods of relief are achieved after successive blocks. However, after a suitable period of conservative management, if radiating pain continues, section of the scalenus anticus muscle should be considered. I prefer to wait for six weeks before considering surgery, since by this time the majority of these patients are relieved by blocks.

Nerve Root Compression Syndrome. A number of patients develop radiation of pain down one or both upper extremities, in the distribution of a nerve root dermatome, a day or two following the initial injury. In most cases, this nerve root compression is related to a traumatic synovitis of the interlaminar joints associated with synovial swelling, which creates pressure upon the nerve root as it passes through the intervertebral foramen (Fig. 66).

Pain. The description of the pain varies from sharp and lancinating to a "pins and needle" sensation. The pain may be aggravated by coughing,

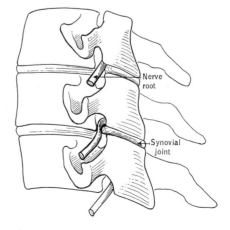

Figure 66. Synovial joint swelling causing nerve root pressure.

97

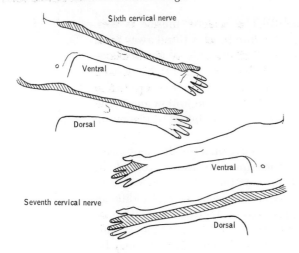

Sixth cervical nerve

Ventral

Dorsal

Ventral

Seventh cervical nerve

Dorsal

Figure 67.   Sixth and seventh cervical root dermatomes.

sneezing, or straining at stool. Movements of the neck frequently produce the pain.

Paresthesia.   Numbness and tingling, if present, occur within the relatively limited geographic area of the nerve root dermatome as compared with the more extensive zone of paresthesia seen with compression of the brachial plexus in the shoulder outlet syndrome. The sixth and seventh cervical nerve roots are most commonly affected (Fig. 67).

Sensation.   If sensory changes are present, they fall within the distribution of the affected nerve roots.

Reflexes.   Reflex changes may or may not be present, depending upon the severity and character of root compression.

Tenderness.   The supraclavicular area is not tender nor are changes reflecting vascular embarrassment apparent.

Treatment of Nerve Root Compression.   Halter cervical traction is usually effective in relieving nerve root compression following an acute cervical strain. In some instances, the 6 to 8 lb. of traction usually used must be increased 2 to 4 lb. to be effective. Ten or 12 pounds of traction is about the limit that a patient wearing a cervical halter can tolerate comfortably for continuous traction. Exceeding this weight causes chafing of the skin, pressure on the mandible with discomfort in the region of the temperomandibular joints, and a variety of other discomforts. When it is important that continuous cervical traction be utilized with much heavier weights, skeletal traction is required, using tongs that attach into the outer table of the skull. By use of these tongs, traction can be maintained at 50 lb. or more without appreciable discomfort. Skeletal traction is ordinarily reserved for fracture dislocations of the cervical spine. If heavier traction is required for acute cervical strain, various types of intermittent halter traction have been designed. These are described in the section on cervical discs (p. 108).

If root compression symptoms persist after subsidence of the acute cervical strain, one must consider the possibility of a herniated cervical disc. After bed rest, traction, physiotherapy, and muscle relaxants have been given an adequate trial, a cervical myelogram should be performed to determine whether a cervical disc is herniated.

Lightheadedness and Vertigo. Since equilibratory symptoms are not appreciated by the patient until he is ambulatory, they usually develop with diminution of the pain, which encourages increased activity. Derangement of the tonic neck-righting reflex is usually considered to be the etiology of this symptom. The spastic cervical musculature is probably sluggish in performing the discrete and imperceptible reflex movements of the head and neck, which act in combination with other centers of equilibrium to maintain balance. A Thomas collar is frequently beneficial in relieving this symptom. This appliance, which immobilizes the neck, probably prevents the deranged neck-righting reflex from playing a part in the function of balance and equilibrium so that this reflex arc is by-passed completely. A corollary to this line of reasoning is the hemispherectomy procedure that is performed on "spastic" children. This operation removes completely the damaged cerebral hemisphere, resulting in improved function of the abnormally innervated limbs. The reason for this improvement is that other lower reflex responses can be substituted for pathologic reflex arcs of a higher order.

Prognosis of Acute Cervical Strain

There is substantial correlation between the age of the patient and the duration of symptoms. Individuals over the age of 60 have a much longer recovery period. Preexisting degenerative arthritic changes of the cervical spine can also be correlated with prolongation of symptoms.

Lengthy litigation is usually accompanied by prolonged symptoms, and settlement of claims is frequently followed by significant improvement in a large percentage of cases. This correlation is of course true to some degree in any pain syndrome involving compensation or litigation.

Neurologic Complications

Occasionally patients who have definite neurologic impairment are admitted through the accident ward with the diagnosis of acute cervical strain or whiplash injury. This impairment may vary from slight motor weakness of the upper or lower extremities to complete quadriplegia. Various entities, such as hematomyelia, acute rupture of a cervical disc, dislocation of the cervical spine, and anterior spinal artery occlusion, must all be considered. Such severe neurologic impairment extends beyond the boundaries of an acute cervical strain and must be treated as an emergency requiring prompt neurologic consultation.

OSTEOARTHRITIS OF THE CERVICAL SPINE

Most patients over 60 years of age have some osteoarthritic changes of the cervical spine, which can be readily identified by x-ray. Since this condition is not in itself a painful condition, for many years it was considered of little or no clinical significance. When these changes occur in the cervical spine, a frequent result is the production of osteophytes or spurs at the vertebral

99

joint spaces in close relationship to the emerging cervical nerve roots. Although osteoarthritis itself is painless, the proximity of the bony changes to the nerve roots gives rise to nerve root compression and cervicobrachial neuralgia.

Pathophysiology

Osteoarthritis is a degenerative condition that is caused by repeated trauma to the joints. The mechanical stress of normal and abnormal motion and weight bearing over the course of many years results in areas of wear or roughening upon the surface of the articular cartilage. This cartilage lacks the capacity to regenerate and to repair defects that arise from the trauma of constant use so that eventully the areas subjected to the greatest stress become completely denuded. The exposed underlying bone becomes eburnated, which literally means converted into an ivory-like mass. This eburnation or osteosclerosis is associated with bony irregularities, particularly at the site of ligamentous attachments and where articulating facets are subjected to strain. Irregularities of the weight bearing surfaces produce poor joint alignment, which places additional stress upon the ligaments and fibrous capsule of the articulating facets. The margins of the vertebral bodies are common sites of exostoses, this so-called "marginal lipping" sometimes extending the entire width of the body. If this lipping occurs on the dorso-lateral portion of the vertebral body, it is called an osteophyte or spur and in this location may cause nerve root compression.

Signs and Symptoms

The symptoms of cervical arthritis are usually gradual in onset and slowly progressive with the passage of time. Most patients are over the age of 60, although it is not exclusively a disease of advanced age. Posterior cervical discomfort is associated with impaired mobility of the cervical spine, particularly extension. The posterior cervical muscles are usually tender and in a variable degree of spasm.

Nerve root compression is manifested by pain extending down the course of the involved dermatome. The radiating pain may be described as aching, burning, tingling, or numbness. The prolonged nerve root pressure may cause motor changes, including muscle weakness, and sometimes perceptible muscle atrophy. Reflex and sensory changes are frequent.

Occasionally, when the osteoarthritic changes are mainly in the form of a prominent median bar or marginal lipping of the dorsal portion of the vertebral body, involvement of the spinal cord occurs. The most common symptom is difficulty in ambulation, which is described by some patients as stiffness and unsteadiness of the lower extremities; others may complain of fatigability and aching of the legs similar to intermittent claudication. Sensory abnormalities involve the upper extremities. This finding is, of course, related to nerve root compression by the same arthritic ridge that also impinges upon the spinal cord. Examination reveals evidence of pyramidal tract damage with hyperactive deep tendon reflexes and extensor plantar responses.

Diagnosis

Osteoarthritis of the cervical cord is readily identified by x-ray. An adequate history and physical examination must be correlated with the x-ray findings. The differential diagnosis must be made between osteoarthritis, scalenus anticus syndrome, and myofascial pain. Aggravation of the pain by movement of the cervical spine, sneezing, coughing, and straining at stool; the progressive history; the typical x-ray picture all aid in clearly defining this condition. Although both scalenus anticus syndrome and myofascial pain offer less of a problem in differential diagnosis than the cervical disc syndrome, it is far less important to differentiate the latter. Since the management of the cervical disc syndrome is similar in most respects to cervical arthritis, the differential is almost academic. Treatment of scalenus anticus syndrome and myofascial pain varies considerably from that of cervical arthritis, and an error in this case results in ineffective treatment.

Treatment

Patients with moderate arthritis of the cervical spine may be adequately managed on an outpatient basis with measures designed to relax muscle spasm. These include heat, gentle massage, and infiltration of local anesthetics, such as procaine or xylocaine.

If the pain is severe and if nerve root compression is present, cervical traction is indicated. In our experience this is best carried out under hospital supervision. The traction should be maintained for as long a period of time as can be tolerated. It is usually necessary to use 8 lb. of traction, which is a bit heavier than that used for cervical muscle spasm. However, this varies according to the size and weight of the patient. Appreciable improvement with halter cervical traction is usually realized within five days if this method is destined to be effective. With improvement, the traction should be maintained for a week to ten days, after which the patient should be quite comfortable. If it appears likely, after several days, that the patient will benefit from traction, he should be measured for a Thomas collar so that when he has improved enough to be ambulated, after a week or ten days, he can wear this appliance whenever he is out of bed. The Thomas collar is beneficial because it helps to maintain the cervical spine in proper position and limits mobility. The collar is worn for six weeks after discharge from the hospital.

Patients with symptoms of nerve root compression who are not benefited by traction should have a cervical myelogram. If a prominent filling defect is revealed by this test and the x-ray findings are in accordance with the clinical picture, surgical decompression of the involved nerve root is indicated. This procedure is described in the discussion on surgery for the cervical disc syndrome (p. 109).

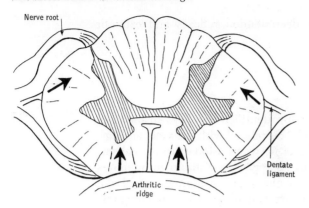

Figure 68. Arthritic ridge causing anterior cord compression and secondary stress upon the cord at the site of attachment of dentate ligament.

Cervical Arthritis and Spinal Cord Compression

Patients who have evidence of spinal cord compression in the presence of cervical arthritis, with or without nerve root symptoms, must be managed from a prophylactic point of view by contrast with most pain problems. Progressive difficulty in ambulation, spasticity of the lower extremities, or sphincter impairment is a firm indication for a cervical myelogram. If complete or partial obstruction from arthritic ridging is seen on myelography, a decompression laminectomy should be performed. In this procedure the bony ridge itself is not usually removed because of the danger of damaging the cervical cord. However, after removal of the spines and lamina, the dura is opened and the dentate ligaments are sectioned at the site of pathologic change. The basis of this procedure is that the spinal cord is firmly fixed by the thin but strong dentate ligaments so that a bony ridge causes symptoms by anterior cord compression with secondary stress upon the cord at the site of attachment of the dentate ligament to the cord (Fig. 68).

THE CERVICAL DISC SYNDROME

Cervical disc disease is inexactly understood by most physicians because of the natural tendency to transpose the mechanisms of the lumbar disc to the cervical region. Although both the cervical and lumbar portions of the spine have fundamental similarities from an anatomic point of view, from a functional or mechanical standpoint they are dissimilar. The lumbar spine is more of a weight bearing structure with limited mobility, while the cervical spine normally furnishes greater mobility in all directions with more minor weight bearing duties. The typical lumbar disc problem is occasionally referred to as a "soft disc" and relates to weight bearing with the degenerated disc herniating out of its normal confines. This soft, degenerated, fibrocartilaginous material, which when removed at surgery resembles nothing more than fragments of crabmeat, is usually the sole cause of nerve root compression. Although an exclusively "soft" cervical disc is seen from time to time, most cervical discs are associated with osteoarthritic changes and are referred to as "hard" discs.

Pathophysiology

Advanced age and repeated mechanical injury, in the form of constant motion and weight bearing, cause degeneration of the cervical intervertebral disc. This degeneration causes the intervertebral disc to lose its normal firm elasticity and to become soft, friable, and granular. The normal intervertebral disc is composed of a soft central portion, called the nucleus pulposus, and the surrounding annulus fibrosus. In the degenerated disc, the nucleus pulposus loses its normal translucent appearance and cannot be differentiated readily from the annulus. The entire disc may eventually become a more or less structureless mass.

Microscopically, there is obliteration of the cellular elements of the disc as the fibers become more scanty and blurred and finally disappear entirely. The completely degenerated disc is seen under the microscope as a diffuse, pink staining hyaline matrix. In addition to these changes, a decrease in the water content of the disc occurs with marked narrowing of the disc. This creates a reduction of its shock absorbing properties so that the increased impact of motion and weight bearing is now transmitted to the vertebral margins and apophyseal joints. Marginal lipping and osteophyte production result from this trauma, creating a combined bony and granular lesion capable of causing spinal cord and nerve root compression.

Because of its position in the curvature of the cervical spine, the interspace between the fifth and sixth cervical vertebrae is by far the most frequent site of involvement with the C4–C5 and C6–C7 interspaces next in order of frequency. The annulus fibrosus, which acts as a retaining ring for the softer nucleus pulposus, is weaker posteriorly; the posterolateral areas are thinner than the central portion, accounting for the tendency of discs to herniate posterolaterally.

At one time it was thought that acute trauma, in the form of a specific blow or accident, was responsible for all ruptured discs. Although trauma is still considered the primary factor in the etiology of these lesions, it is believed that this is in the form of chronic trauma in which a lifetime of normal and abnormal movements of the head and neck cause degenerative changes. Acute trauma may, however, precipitate symptoms in the presence of preexisting degenerative changes.

Signs and Symptoms

The patient with cervical disc disease usually gives a history of occasional "stiff necks" for some years. Initially these symptoms are usually lightly dismissed as related to a cool draft of air or some strenuous activity. With the passage of time this intermittent stiff neck becomes an almost constant ache in the posterior cervical region. By the time the cervical pain has assumed proportions that awake concern in the patient, nerve root com-

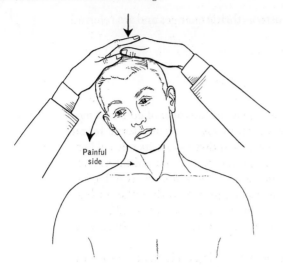

Figure 69. Foraminal compression test.

Painful side

pression symptoms are often present. This may first be manifested as pain in the shoulder, and next in the arm, until the entire nerve root dermatome is involved, extending into the hand. The nerve root pain is usually constant but varies in intensity from an intense discomfort to a hardly perceptible paresthesia. The nature of the pain may vary from a dull ache to sharp, lancinating, electric-like stabs. The entire course of the involved dermatome may not be involved and frequently a large segment is "skipped" so that the pain is appreciated in the shoulder and upper arm and then not again until the hand and fingers become involved. Coughing, sneezing, straining, or changes in position of the cervical spine may aggravate the pain, particularly radicular or nerve root pain. Sensory phenomena, in the form of numbness or paresthesia, are frequent and follow the involved dermatome.

Atrophy, weakness, and muscle fasciculations within the involved myotome may be seen in long-standing cases. Sensory examination usually reveals some sensory impairment of the involved dermatome. Reflex changes vary according to the specific nerve root involved. Movements of the cervical spine should be performed carefully and gently. Hyperextension and lateral and anterior flexion may all be painful and reproduce the radiating pain. The foraminal compression test in which the head and neck are titled toward the painful side while pressure is applied to the top of the head frequently reproduces the radicular symptoms (Fig. 69).

Diagnosis

X-ray Changes. A history and physical findings typical of cervical disc disease are usually corroborated by x-ray changes in the cervical spine. The lateral views reveal:

1. Narrowing of the involved intervertebral disc space.
2. Osteoarthritic changes particularly involving the vertebral bodies adjacent to the narrowed interspace.

3. Straightening of the normal lordotic cervical curvature.

The oblique views frequently reveal the presence of osteophytes within the intervertebral foramina, which may be most marked on the side and level of suspected pathology.

Dermatomes.   In numbering the interspaces, radiologists are prone to refer to the lower vertebral body. By this system, the space between the fifth and sixth cervical vertebrae becomes the C6 interspace. I have also encountered physicians who are in the habit of referring to the upper vertebral body in referring to the disc space. Surgery mistakenly performed one interspace above or below the site of actual disease is not likely to produce a fortunate result, and I can only condemn this ambiguous method of nomenclature. The interspace between the fifth and sixth cervical vertebrae is properly referred to as the C5-C6 interspace.

C5-C6 Disc Disease.   The most common site of cervical disc disease is the C5-C6 interspace (Fig. 70). This particular disc space is the area of greatest mechanical activity in the cervical spine from the point of view of both

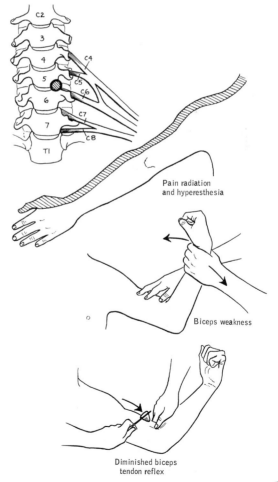

Figure 70.   Signs and symptoms of C5-C6 disc disease.

105

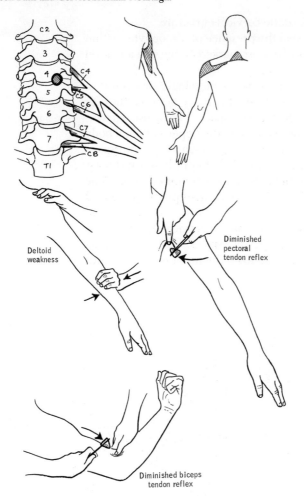

Deltoid
weakness

Diminished
pectoral
tendon reflex

Diminished biceps
tendon reflex

Figure 71. Signs and symptoms of C4-C5 disc disease.

movement and weight bearing. The C5-C6 disc causes involvement of the sixth cervical nerve root. Pain radiation and hypesthesia involve the dermatome of the sixth cervical nerve root. If motor weakness is present, it is usually the biceps muscle that demonstrates this weakness. The biceps tendon reflex is diminished on the painful side.

C4-C5 Disc Disease. Next in order of frequency in cervical disc disease is the C4-C5 interspace, which causes involvement of the C5 nerve root (Fig. 71). Pain radiation and hypesthesia involve the dermatome of the fifth cervical nerve root. The deltoid muscle best demonstrates motor weakness if present. Reflex changes may be demonstrated in both the pectoral and biceps reflexes.

C6-C7 Disc Disease. Of the three most common sites of cervical disc disease, the C6-C7 interspace is the least common, causing involvement of the C7 nerve root (Fig. 72). Pain radiation and hypesthesia involve the dermatome of the seventh cervical nerve root. Motor weakness of the triceps muscle may be present. The triceps reflex is diminished.

Management

Approximately 80 per cent of all patients with cervical disc disease can be adequately managed by conservative therapy. All patients with an attack of cervical disc disease should be placed at bed rest. Aspirin in doses of 10 gr. (0.6 gm.) every four hours in conjunction with muscle relaxants may be adequate to relieve the symptoms. If these measures are not sufficient to relieve pain, the patient should be hospitalized for cervical traction. This is most effective with the patient at absolute bed rest, using 6 to to 8 lb. of traction weight. The use of muscle relaxants in conjunction with cervical traction augments the effectiveness of the traction. In addition to the muscle relaxing properties of the drug, a sedative side effect is frequently obtained, which helps reduce the natural restlessness of the patient who is undergoing a confining and rather uncomfortable treatment.

Occasionally the results of cervical halter traction may not be completely satisfactory. It is possible that the amount of traction weight that can be brought into play by continuous cervical traction is not sufficient. It is difficult for the patient to tolerate much more than 8 or 10 lb. of continuous

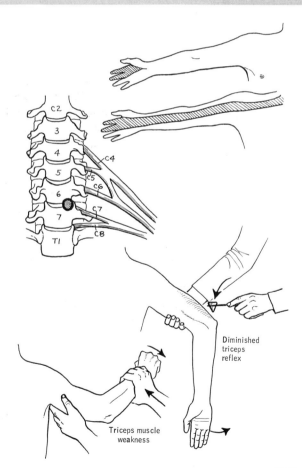

Figure 72. Signs and symptoms of C6-C7 disc disease.

107

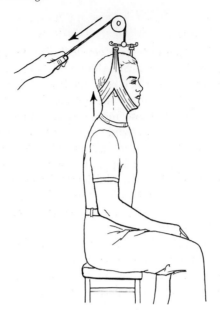

Figure 73.   Sayre traction.

traction. However, much greater loads can be tolerated for short intervals. One method of intermittent cervical traction is Sayre traction, which consists of the patient's sitting in a chair or standing, while by means of overhead halter and pulley arrangement he is actually lifted off his feet for short periods of time (Fig. 73). Dr. Sayre, who introduced this apparatus in 1850, was mainly interested in a device that would support the patient during the application of a plaster jacket. Its therapeutic values were quickly realized, and today some modification of the Sayre traction apparatus is standard equipment in every physical medicine department. Although this is an effective method of traction, it is usually used for limited intervals of time, since the patient in most instances is transported from his room to the physiotherapy department for the treatment, and a therapist is required in attendance.

Intermittent mechanical cervical traction has the advantage of prolonged intervals of application, since it can be carried out in the patient's room with the patient at bed rest. The apparatus constructed for this purpose exerts by means of an electric motor an adjustable traction force for a minute or two, followed by a traction-free period of a minute. These traction-free intervals, although short, are extremely important, since they allow the patient to tolerate "pulls" of 30 lb. or more for prolonged periods of time.

After several weeks of conservative management, both at home and in the hospital, if the patient continues to have severe pain, cervical myelography should be considered.

This x-ray study consists of performing a lumbar puncture and introducing 9 cc. of Pantopaque, a radiopaque substance, into the subarachnoid space. With patient upon an x-ray tilt-table, the radiologist can control the flow of the dye column so that any segment of the spine can be studied.

Pantopaque, which has an oily consistency, is heavier than spinal fluid, and it is necessary to tilt the head of the table down in order to visualize the cervical spine. The cerebral ventricles communicate directly with the spinal subarachnoid space, making it possible for the Pantopaque to spill over into the cerebral ventricles if the x-ray table is tilted excessively. This is to be avoided, since once the dye is within the ventricles it cannot be removed readily. After the cervical myelogram has been performed, by reversing the tilt of the x-ray table the Pantopaque is brought back to the lumbar region and collected in the vicinity of the spinal needle, which is usually left in place during the procedure. The radiopaque material is then removed through the needle by gently aspirating with a 10 cc. syringe. If a significant and constant filling defect is demonstrated by myelography, surgery is considered.

Cervical Disc Surgery

Probably the most important single factor affecting the outcome of cervical disc surgery is surgical technique. This concept may well be at variance with

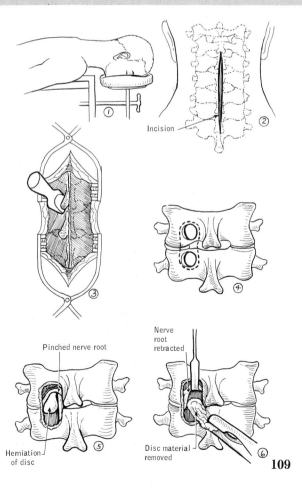

Figure 74. (1) Patient positioned with cervical spine straightened or slightly flexed. (2) Midline incision. (3)A unilateral subperiosteal muscle dissection is performed. (4) The best way to afford maximal exposure of the nerve root and minimal exposure of the cord is to perform the laminectomy laterally. This is accomplished by connecting two laterally placed burr holes in adjacent laminae. (5) Exposure of disc responsible for nerve root compression. (6) Removal of disc material.

Incision

Pinched nerve root

Herniation of disc

Nerve root retracted

Disc material removed

109

the general opinion, since physicians often believe that the judgment exercised in selecting candidates for surgery is the cardinal issue. Variations in surgical technique do not play so great a role in lumbar disc disease, which is as a rule less difficult to manage than cervical problems.

The various steps involving a cervical hemilaminectomy and removal of a disc are illustrated in Fig. 74. It is of prime importance to carry the hemilaminectomy laterally to provide complete exposure of the nerve root. This not only facilitates the exposure in removing the herniated disc but serves as a foraminotomy to decompress the swollen nerve root. In most instances a bony spur can be found at the site of the protruded disc. Unless this bony projection is unusually large, it is not necessary to remove it with a chisel or dental burr if a thorough foraminotomy has been performed to decompress the root.

SCALENUS ANTICUS SYNDROME

Scalenus anticus syndrome is the term used to designate brachial plexus compression neuralgia caused by pressure of the anterior scalene muscle with or without a cervical rib. Some physicians label the cervical rib syndrome and the scalenus anticus syndrome as two distinct entities, thereby creating an arbitrary classification of no clinical value, since the signs, symptoms, and treatment are the same for both.

Pathophysiology

The scalenus anticus muscle arises by tendinous attachments from the transverse processes of the third to the sixth cervical vertebrae and is inserted on the superior surface of the first rib. The scalenus medius muscle originates from the posterior tubercles of the third to seventh cervical vertebrae and inserts upon the upper surface of the first rib. A triangle is formed with the rib as a base, the scalenus medius behind, and the scalenus anticus muscle in front. The subclavian artery and the brachial plexus arch over the first rib behind the insertion of the scalenus anticus muscle and pass downward to the arm (Fig. 75). Posterior to the nerves and vessel is the scalenus medius muscle. The structures within this triangle are susceptible to pressure produced by abnormal forces encroaching upon this already snug space.

Spasm or hypertrophy of the scalenus anticus muscle is frequently cited as the cause of compression of the structures within the "shoulder outlet triangle." It is not clear whether spasm of this muscle creates its effect by elevating the first rib to which it is attached or by developing an abnormally wide and thick attachment to the rib and causing a diminution of the scalene triangle.

A common congenital anomaly is the cervical rib, a supernumerary rib, which usually originates from the seventh cervical vertebra on one or both sides (Fig. 76). This bony prominence may thrust the scalenus medius muscle forward against the scalenus anticus muscle, which significantly

110

diminishes the space within the scalene triangle and produces compression of its contents. This anomaly is often present without clinical symptoms and is frequently discovered by an x-ray of the chest or cervical spine obtained for an unrelated problem. The size and configuration of this bony prominence vary from an enlarged transverse process on the seventh cervical vertebra to a completely formed rib possessed of a true cartilage that unites with the cartilage of the first rib.

Individuals with bilateral cervical ribs frequently present symptoms on one side only—usually the right side in right handed people. This implies that an anatomic variant must be augmented by additional factors before symptoms appear. This point is also borne out by the usual occurrence of this syndrome in middle age even though the anatomic structures have been present since birth.

One of the stigmas of middle age is the frequent deterioration of good posture, causing the thoracic cage to sag a bit and increasing the pull upon the scalene muscles. The increased tension upon these muscles reduces the

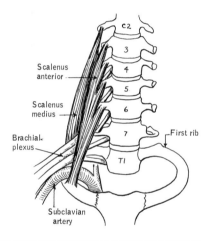

Figure 75. The structures comprising the scalenus anticus triangle.

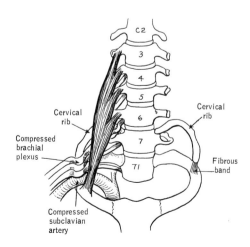

Figure 76. Cervical rib causing brachial plexus and subclavian artery compression.

111

available space within the scalene triangle and causes compression of the brachial plexus and the subclavian artery.

Trauma is frequently cited as a precipitant of the scalenus anticus syndrome. This is usually an indirect injury, such as an acute cervical strain or whiplash, which frequently causes severe spasm of the scalene muscles and the posterior cervical muscle groups.

Cervical disc disease associated with nerve root compression may cause a secondary scalenus anticus syndrome by reflex spasm of the scalenus anticus muscle due to irritation of the cervical nerve roots.

Signs and Symptoms

Almost all patients with scalenus anticus syndrome complain of persistent pain extending into the upper extremity. The pain is often described as dull and aching, but such descriptions as sharp, knife-like, or electric shock-like may also be elicited. Radiation of the pain may occur down the forearm into the hand along either the ulnar or radial aspect, or sometimes both, depending on the extent and position of compression upon the brachial plexus. Discomfort of a rather vague and general nature is frequently appreciated in the supraclavicular area, sometimes extending into the posterior cervical region. Frequently any strenuous activity involving the painful arm aggravates the pain. Routine household duties, such as sweeping, dusting, washing, and mowing the lawn, may be cited as precipitating the pain. In some patients the position of the involved extremity assumes greater significance than the amount of motor activity. Elevation of the extremities for prolonged periods of time often initiates an attack of pain.

A housewife who came under our care had never experienced pain, in spite of a routinely strenuous round of daily activities, until she attempted to paint the walls of a small room. This task necessitated the elevation of her right upper extremity for rather prolonged periods and was followed by a very severe scalenus anticus syndrome. Once the syndrome had been precipitated, it subsequently could be "triggered" by any strenuous activity of the involved extremity. We recently encountered a truck driver who had been considered neurotic by several physicians because of the seemingly bizarre nature of his symptoms. He reported pain in both upper extremities only when driving the truck but had no discomfort when he drove his own car. The truck he drove was a model featuring an unusually high, flat steering wheel, which he was accustomed to drive with his forearms resting on the wheel. The combination of the high steering wheel and his habitual position when driving caused an unusual degree of upper extremity elevation, which was not present when he drove an ordinary car.

A neurosurgeon in Philadelphia found that whenever he performed a cervical laminectomy with the patient in the sitting position, requiring prolonged elevation of his upper extremities, he developed mild symptoms of scalenus anticus syndrome on the right side. He now performs the procedure with the patient prone. Many other occupations and avocations also require prolonged elevation of the upper extremities. We have treated school teachers who write on blackboards, auto mechanics, trap shooters, food servers in cafeterias, traffic policemen, and many others who could associate their symptoms with prolonged elevation of the upper extremities.

If symptoms persist for a prolonged period, motor weakness eventually progressing to muscle atrophy may occur. Sensory impairment may vary from mild hypesthesia to complete anesthesia. Decreased reflexes are sometimes found.

Vascular symptoms occur in some cases and may be due to pressure irritation of the sympathetic innervation to the limb, which follows the medial cord of the brachial plexus and the subclavian artery, or it may be related to direct pressure upon the subclavian artery causing partial occlusion of the vessel. Symptoms of sympathetic irritation may resemble Raynaud's phenomenon. The hand becomes stiff and slightly swollen; the skin assumes a glossy appearance and is often perceptibly cooler to the touch than the uninvolved hand. Sometimes a dusky coloration can be seen in the affected hand. When direct arterial occlusion is present, the radial pulse is diminished and at times imperceptible, depending on the degree of circulatory embarrassment. We have treated three cases of thrombosis of the subclavian artery resulting from the prolonged compression of a hypertrophied scalenus anticus muscle. When this occurs, the blood pressure of the involved extremity is low or occasionally unobtainable, and trophic changes may progress to digital gangrene.

Diagnosis

A patient with a history of cervicobrachial neuralgia, affected by positional changes of the upper extremity, requires evaluation for a possible scalenus anticus syndrome. The routine examination includes testing for sensory impairment and muscle weakness and examination for signs of vascular embarrassment to the affected extremity. Careful attention is given to the supraclavicular area, which is palpated carefully to detect any abnormal fullness or prominence that could be due to a cervical rib or hypertrophied scalenus anticus muscle. Pressure over the region of the scalenus anticus muscle is invariably associated with tenderness in the presence of a scalenus anticus syndrome, and frequently this maneuver causes radiation of pain down the affected extremity.

The radial pulse is carefully palpated and the two sides compared. Several classic maneuvers designed to increase the preexisting compression upon the subclavian artery may cause temporary obliteration of the radial pulse. These tests are useful but must be interpreted with caution and in relationship to the history and physical findings, since obliteration of the radial pulse can be caused by these maneuvers in many individuals not affected with scalenus anticus syndrome.

Allen Maneuver. With the forearm flexed at a 90 degree angle, the arm is extended horizontally and rotated externally at the shoulder; the head is rotated so that the chin is pointed toward the opposite shoulder (Fig. 77).

Adson Maneuver. The extremity to be tested is maintained in a dependent position; the head is rotated so that the chin is pointed at the ipsilateral shoulder. The patient is instructed to take a deep inspiration and maintain it while the radial pulse is palpated (Fig. 78).

Halstead Maneuver. Downward traction is maintained upon the tested extremity while the neck is hyperextended and the head is rotated toward the contralateral shoulder (Fig. 79).

As part of the routine evaluation of every cervicobrachial neuralgia, x-rays of the cervical spine are obtained to determine the presence of a cervical rib or cervical spine disease.

Infiltration of the scalenus anticus muscle with a local anesthetic is considered by some physicians to be the diagnostic test of greatest value. In such a diagnostic infiltration, no more than 2 or 3 cc. of solution are injected in an effort to limit the anesthesia to the muscle and avoid involvement of the brachial plexus or sympathetic chain, which may produce relief of pain unrelated to relaxation of the muscle. In our experience, this diagnostic block is

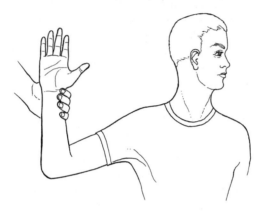

Figure 77. Allen maneuver.

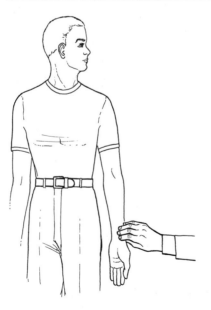

Figure 78. Adson maneuver.

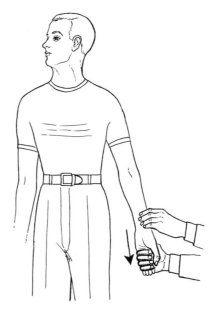

Figure 79. Halstead maneuver.

not completely reliable. It is a helpful aid but one that must be fitted into the general medical pattern of the syndrome.

The greatest problem in differential diagnosis of this syndrome is the cervicobrachial pains of cervical nerve root compression due to arthritis of the cervical spine or to cervical disc disease. Nerve root pain may be aggravated by coughing, sneezing, or straining at stool and is less affected by positional changes of the involved extremity. X-ray of the cervical spine may be helpful in determining the existence of cervical disease. In some cases, when the differential is difficult, it may be necessary to perform a cervical myelogram to completely rule out involvement of the spine. We have, on occasion, had patients with neoplasm of the superior pulmonary sulcus (Pancoast's tumor) whose admitting diagnosis was scalenus anticus syndrome; this emphasizes the importance of a chest x-ray in the routine work-up of this syndrome. Raynaud's disease is usually not too difficult to differentiate. The symptoms are usually bilateral with the characteristic history of cold causing the hands and fingers to undergo color changes.

Treatment

Conservative treatment consists of infiltration of the scalenus anticus muscle in an attempt to eliminate the immediate cause of pressure and postural correction in an effort to reduce the underlying cause of the problem.

Infiltration Technique. The procedure is performed with the patient seated (Fig. 80). With the head in a neutral position the clavicular insertion of the sternocleidomastoid muscle is palpated and pushed medially with the middle finger of the left hand. The patient is instructed to breathe deeply, and the scalenus anticus muscle can be felt just posterior to the middle finger

115

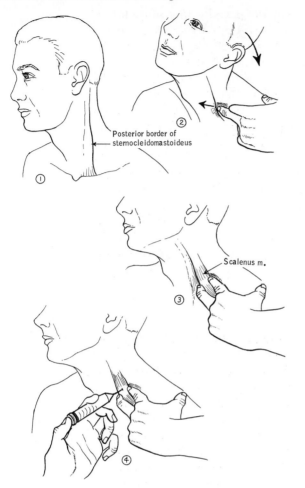

Posterior border of
sternocleidomastoideus

Scalenus m.

Figure 80. Technique of infiltrating spastic scalenus anterior muscle.

as a firm, thick cord, which tightens with each inspiration. The scalenus muscle is then straddled with the middle and index fingers of the left hand and the head tilted away from the side to be injected. The injection of local anesthetic directly into the muscle belly is carried out with a needle no longer than one inch. Once scalenus anticus muscle relaxation is achieved with infiltration of local anesthetic, relief of pain may persist for periods far in excess of the effect of the block.

Correction of poor posture, in addition to correction of a sagging stance, also involves weight reduction in obese patients and alleviation of any special problems, such as the use of proper support for pendulous breasts. The patient is often benefited by sleeping on two or three pillows and occasionally by sleeping with a pillow beneath the involved shoulder.

Surgery

If conservative methods are not effective, surgery is indicated. The tendinous insertion of the scalenus anticus muscle is divided just above the first rib, regardless of the presence of a cervical rib. Usually this procedure is adequate to decompress the brachial plexus and subclavian artery, and as soon as all the muscle fibers are divided, the subclavian artery and the lower trunk of the brachial plexus will slide forward and be free within the supraclavicular triangle. If the vessel and nerves remain compressed by the cervical rib, a resection of the bony anomaly is then carried out.

Technique (Fig. 81). (1) The patient is placed in supine position with the neck slightly extended and the head rotated toward the opposite shoulder. An incision is made a thumbsbreadth above and parallel to the clavicle, starting over the clavicular insertion of the sternocleidomastoid muscle and carried laterally about 8 cm. (2) The platysma muscle is divided, exposing the tendon of the sternocleidomastoid muscle with its attachment to the clavicle. (3) The clavicular portion of the sternocleidomastoid muscle is divided, exposing the omohyoid muscle, which is also divided. At this point, the scalenus anticus muscle, which is stretched taut by the position of the head and neck, can easily be palpated as a firm bundle of muscle fibers.

Figure 81. Technique of scalenotomy. (Numbers refer to steps outlined in text.)

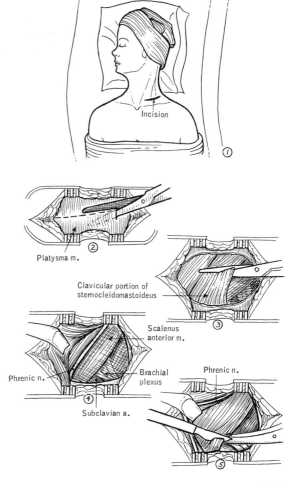

(4) The fat and fascia overlying the scalenus anticus muscle are carefully dissected to identify the phrenic nerve, which runs obliquely across the muscle from the lateral to the medial border. When this procedure is carried out on the left side, the fatty tissue above and medial to the scalenus anticus muscle is retracted medially with the phrenic nerve to avoid injury to the thoracic duct. (5) A knife or scissors is used to divide the musculotendinous insertion of the muscle in small groups of fibers, which retract upward as they are sectioned, exposing the uncut fibers. When the muscle is completely divided, the arch of the subclavian artery and the lower trunk of the brachial plexus can be visualized and are seen to be free.

If a prominent cervical rib can be seen to cause further compression of these structures, this bony anomaly must be resected. The rib is carefully palpated and the subclavian artery and trunks of the brachial plexus carefully identified to avoid injury to these structures. The fascia and periosteum are incised over the most prominent portion of the rib. A careful subperiosteal dissection is carried out, using a periosteal elevator. When the rib is stripped of periosteum as far as possible, a rongeur is used to remove the bone piecemeal.

When all bleeding has been carefully controlled and the wound is to be closed, the anesthetist may remove the sandbag, producing extension of the neck, and bring the head into neutral position to facilitate closure by relaxing the muscles. The omohyoid and the divided fibers of the sternocleidomastoid are sutured, using mattress sutures of chromic catgut. The subcutaneous and skin layers are closed, using interrupted black silk technique. No drain is used.

chapter six

Low Back Pain and Sciatica

chapter six –

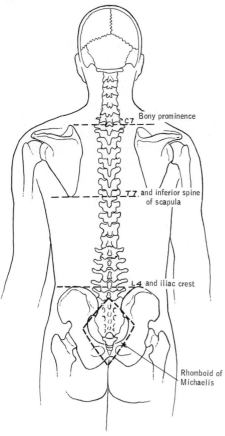

Figure 82.   Significant surface landmarks readily identified on routine examination of the back.

Low Back Pain and Sciatica

Low back pain in all probability causes more general discomfort than any other medical problem except the common cold. It has been estimated that every year 250,000 workers in the United States incur low back injuries while at work for which they take time off from their job and receive financial compensation. Many of these individuals are incapacitated for longer periods than workers who have suffered more conspicuous injuries, such as fractured limbs or severe lacerations. Thus, in terms of time lost from work and compensation payments, low back pain is one of the nation's costliest symptoms. The available statistics for industrial accidents is probably only the apparent part of the picture, for an uncounted host of housewives and white collar workers may not report their symptoms.

The objective findings in many types of low back pain are often random, uncertain, and open to varied interpretations. This is true not only of the physical findings but also of the x-ray interpretation. Some radiologists estimate that approximately one quarter of the lumbosacral spines subjected to x-ray study reveal some abnormality. Frequently the patient with a very obvious x-ray abnormality may never experience any low back discomfort, while the possessor of a spine that appears normal radiographically can hardly hobble about. Unfortunately this unreliability of diagnostic findings lends itself to litigation in which the plaintiff claims severe and permanent incapacitation while the defense is hard at work minimizing the injury.

Of course the basis of all the difficulty experienced in the low back region is the tremendous work load concentrated in this relatively small area. Whenever an individual straightens up from a bent-over position, he is utilizing his lumbosacral spine as a fulcrum, which concentrates a force of over a quarter of a ton within the lower lumbar and sacral regions. If an object is lifted from the bent-over position, the weight of the object can be multiplied by a leverage factor of 12 to 16, depending upon the length of the torso and the position of the arms. Thus, the frail housewife who bends forward to pick up her small child can subject her lumbosacral spine to a stress of as much as half a ton or more. The increasingly sedentary habits of our population are undoubtedly a factor in the generally increasing problem of low back pain. This creates a situation in which the lower back must be able to tolerate tremendous loads without the slightest preparation. The office worker who must struggle with a jammed window and the typist and her roommate who must move a heavy sofa in cleaning their apartment are indiscreetly gambling that their sedentary ligaments and tissues will support these sudden and unexpected loads.

STRUCTURE AND MECHANICS OF THE LOWER BACK

It is somewhat the fashion for those who discuss the ills of the lower back to start with our antecedents, who allegedly crawled out of the ocean to develop eventually into man who assumed the upright position. The basic thesis is that the architecture of the trunk and the spine is not yet adjusted to the upright position and that many of the difficulties suffered in this area are related to lack of complete structural adaptation. I believe that the back is

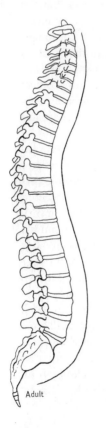

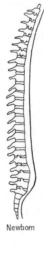

Newborn

Adult

Figure 83. The normal curves of the spine vary according to age.

constructed about as well as any of the other major segments and organs of the body, and, like the heart subjected to a high fat diet or the stomach responding to emotional and gastric abuses, the back usually will give way if treated improperly. The individual who travels to his place of employment by car, uses the elevator to deliver him to his office, sits behind a desk all day, and returns home to immobilize himself in upholstered furniture gazing at television every evening cannot expect his tissues to sustain him in a strenuous tennis match on the weekend.

Several significant surface landmarks are readily identified on routine examination of the back (Fig. 82). At the base of the cervical spine the midline prominence of the spinous processes of the seventh cervical and first thoracic vertebrae may be seen and palpated. In thin individuals the outlines of the scapula can be palpated and the inferior angle of this bone is opposite the seventh thoracic vertebra. The iliac crests can usually be palpated to reveal the level of the fourth lumbar vertebra. The top of the sacroiliac joint is at the level of the third sacral vertebra.

The angulation of the spinous processes is acute in the thoracic region so that the tip of each spinous process lies over the body of the next inferior vertebra. This angulation decreases in the lumbar region so that the tip of each lumbar spinous process lies over the inferior margin of the same vertebral body. In children, the spinal cord ends at the space between the third and fourth lumbar vertebrae, but as the child increases in size, the end of the cord gradually ascends to terminate at the lower border of the first lumbar vertebra.

The normal curves of the spine vary according to age (Fig. 83). The spine of the newborn presents a thoracic curve extending from the second to the twelfth thoracic vertebrae and a sacral curve coinciding with the sacrum and coccyx. Both these curves bend concavely forward and develop during intrauterine life as accommodation curves for the thoracic and pelvic viscera. When the infant is able to sit upright at about three months of age, the cervical curve starts to develop. This curvature extends from the atlas to the second thoracic vertebra and bends convexly forward. When the child begins to walk, about the end of the first year, the lumbar curve starts to form but is not consolidated until adult life. This curve extends from the twelfth thoracic vertebra to the sacrum and bends convexly forward. These secondary or acquired curves neutralize the primary or accommodation curves, allow the spine to transmit the weight of the trunk to the pelvis almost completely by bony support, and reduce the muscular effort needed to maintain the erect posture. In females, the lumbar curve, which is more pronounced than in males, undergoes flattening during pregnancy, but the normal anterior convexity is restored rapidly after delivery.

The vertebral column consists of 33 vertebrae joined together by multiple ligaments and intervening cartilages. Each vertebra is composed of a body, which has a weight bearing function, and a neural arch with its accessory processes, which, in addition to protecting the spinal cord, provide attachment sites for muscles and ligaments (Fig. 84). The weight borne by each vertebra increases progressively downward, and this is reflected in the increasingly more massive vertebral bodies seen in the descent from the cervical to the lumbar regions. The intervertebral discs are constructed

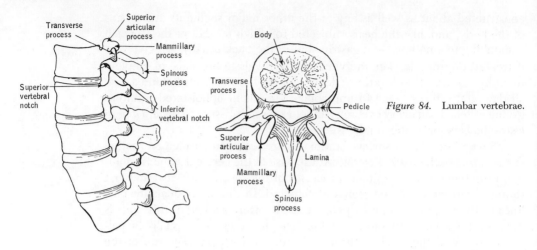

Figure 84. Lumbar vertebrae.

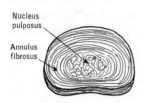

Figure 85. Intervertebral disc.

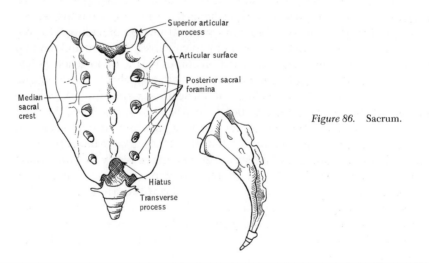

Figure 86. Sacrum.

primarily for weight bearing and motion and, like the vertebrae, they become larger as they go progressively downward. These structures are composed of the annulus fibrosus, made up of concentric layers of connective tissue fibers, and the nucleus pulposus, a spongy, viscous, central mass of fibrocartilage (Fig. 85). The main function of the annulus fibrosus is to confine and pre-

124

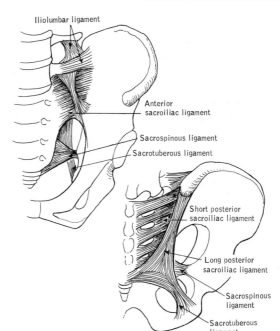

Figure 87. Sacroiliac ligaments.

serve the shape of the nucleus pulposus, but it also aids in holding the vertebrae together. The nucleus pulposus, by virtue of its soft consistency, maintains the transmission of forces uniformly over the entire surface of the vertebral body and in this manner behaves as a shock absorber.

The sacrum is a large wedge shaped bone representing the developmental fusion of its five vertebral segments (Fig. 86). Its superior surface is oval and articulates with the inferior aspect of the body of the fifth lumbar vertebra. The lower portion of the sacrum articulates with the coccyx, which is made up of four rudimentary vertebrae.

The sacrum is wedged into the pelvis and is the keystone between the vertebral column and the lower extremities. The sacroiliac joints are formed by the lateral portions of the sacrum and the articular surface of the ilium. A joint capsule is attached to the margins of the articular surfaces, and the bones are held together by the anterior sacroiliac, long posterior sacroiliac, short posterior sacroiliac, and interosseous ligaments (Fig. 87).

Low Back Musculature

There are not many muscles whose prime function is support and movement of the lower back. However, there are a number of muscle groupings that originate or insert within the low back region lending support and augmenting movement of the lower back as a secondary function.

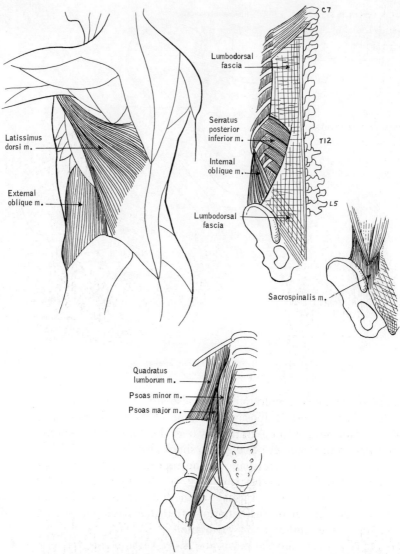

Figure 88. Low back musculature.

The following muscles are directly related to movement of the low back region (Fig. 88):

Latissimus dorsi

> *Origin.* Spinous processes of six lower dorsal and lumbar and sacral vertebrae, crest of ilium, and four lowest ribs.

> *Insertion.* Bicipital groove of humerus.

External oblique

> *Origin.* Eight lowest ribs.

> *Insertion.* Crest of ilium, Poupart's ligament, crest of pubis.

Sacrospinalis

> *Origin.* Dorsal surface of sacrum, spines of lumbar vertebrae, crest of ilium.

Insertion. Divides into iliocostalis and longissimus dorsi, oocupying the groove along the spinous processes from the sacrum to the neck.

Internal oblique

Origin. Crest of ilium, Poupart's ligament, and lumbar fascia.

Insertion. Six lowest ribs, linea alba, crest of pubis.

Serratus posterior inferior

Origin. Spines of lower two thoracic and upper three lumbar vertebrae.

Insertion. Four lower ribs.

Quadratus lumborum

Origin. Crest of ilium and transverse processes of third, fourth, and fifth lumbar vertebrae.

Insertion. Twelfth rib and transverse processes of third, fourth, and fifth lumbar vertebrae.

Psoas major

Origin. Last dorsal and all lumbar vertebrae.

Insertion. Lesser trochanter of femur.

The lumbodorsal fascia is a thick investing membrane covering the deep muscles of the back of the trunk and continuing upward through the thoracic region to the base of the neck. Inferiorly, it is attached to the iliac crest and to the distal and lateral margins of the sacrum and its spines. In the lumbar and thoracic regions, it is attached to the spinous processes of the vertebrae.

EXAMINATION OF THE LOWER BACK

The great variety of conditions that may be related to low back pain necessitates a most careful history. In taking the history, the following questions must be answered:

1. Did the pain occur after injury or unusual physical exertion, or did it develop spontaneously?

2. Where is the pain, and does it extend or radiate?

3. What factors aggravate and relieve the pain?

4. Has the pain improved or worsened since its onset?

In addition to these questions, which are specifically concerned with the pain, the following secondary points must be covered before the problem can be properly evaluated: First, the medical history should include a review of previous hospitalizations. This information may furnish insight into specific psychologic tendencies as well as rounding out the general, overall, medical picture. For example, was the patient hospitalized for vague gastrointestinal complaints on one occasion and again for vague chest pains and were the studies performed in both these hospital stays negative? Second, a history of multiple surgical procedures should ring a warning bell in the mind of the examiner. Third, is litigation anticipated or is the amount of compensation to be received likely to be an issue?

If a systematic routine is followed in examining the back, all important areas will be covered in a brief period of time. Since the patient must be examined sitting, standing, prone, and supine, a natural sequence should be established that will not force the patient to hop repeatedly on and off the

127

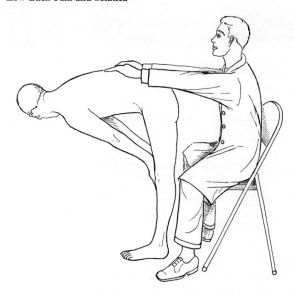

Figure 89. Mobility of the lumbar spine is tested by having the patient bend forward and by observing and palpating the changes in the lumbar curvature.

examining table and to assume the same position several times during the course of the examination. Not only is it needlessly time consuming, but this lack of an orderly approach makes it more difficult to evaluate a case properly.

The examination of the back should begin the instant the patient enters the office. Often a great deal can be learned by observing him walk the short distance to a chair and sit down while he is not self-conscious about being scrutinized. During the taking of history it is well to note how uncomfortable he is and any unusual features about his stance or carriage. When examining men, I usually take the concluding portion of the history in the examining room while they are removing their clothing so that I may observe how these movements are performed. An adequate low back examination can be accomplished if patients are allowed to retain their underwear.

The back is inspected with the patient standing. The normal median depression starts just below the hairline and extends to the sacrum. Any marked lateral curvature of the spine will be closely followed by this median depression. The prominence of the seventh cervical and the first thoracic vertebrae is easily noted, and in thin persons the spaced elevations representing the spinous processes of the vertebrae can be seen descending to the sacrum. A diamond shaped area over the sacrum can be identified in individuals with good muscular development (see Fig. 82). This is the rhomboid of Michaelis, formed by the dimples at the posterior superior spines of the ilium, the lines formed by the gluteal muscles, and the groove at the lower end of the spine. Normally the vertical axis of this rhomboid is parallel with the long axis of the body. The gluteal creases are examined and should be on the same level. A loss of the normal lumbar curvature is usually seen as a somewhat flattened lumbar area.

Palpation of the lumbar and lower thoracic regions is performed on either side of the midline in an effort to determine the presence of spasm of the paraspinal musculature. The iliac crests are palpated and inspected to determine whether they are of equal height.

The examiner places his hand on the patient's lumbar spine, and the patient is asked to bend forward, backward, and to either side (Fig. 89). Normally an evenly distributed curve of the lumbar spine accompanies each of these movements. The degree of total body mobility is not of prime importance. Some individuals with a completely immobile lumbar spine can actually touch their toes by compensating for the lack of lumbar mobility with hypermobility of the hips and the remaining vertebrae. For this reason, during the performance of these maneuvers, the palpating hand is placed on the back to determine impairment in any particular segment of the spine. Tenderness to palpation in any specific area of the low back is noted. Atrophy and loss of tone of the muscles of the thigh and calf can best be evaluated in the standing position.

The patient is then asked to kneel on a chair with his feet projecting several inches beyond the edge of the seat. This is the optimal position for obtaining the ankle jerks; one side is compared with the other (Fig. 90). The patient is then asked to sit on the edge of the examining table with his legs hanging over the edge of the table. This is the best position for obtaining the knee jerks, both of which are compared (Fig. 91).

The patient is then asked to lie on his back on the examining table. In this position the lower extremities are measured as follows: The circumference of the thighs and calves is measured six inches above and below the middle of the patella. The length of the legs is measured from the anterior superior iliac spine to the medial malleolus.

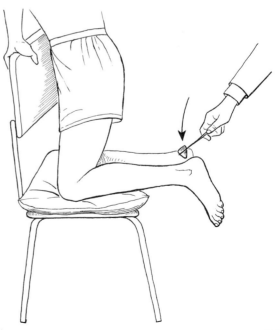

Figure 90. The Achilles reflex is best elicited where the patient is in the kneeling position.

The sensation of the lower extremities is tested with a pin. In performing a sensory examination, it is not necessary to hurt the patient with the pin; in fact, a painful session may often lessen the patient's cooperation. Since the physician is looking for nerve root compression with numbness in a specific dermatome, each dermatome is tested and compared with that of the opposite side.

Testing for possible weakness of the toe extensors and flexors is performed with the patient in the supine position. In most cases, when one is concerned with single root compression symptoms, such as would occur from a herniated disc, testing such smaller muscle groupings is frequently helpful, whereas testing the larger muscles proves of diagnostic benefit less often. The extensors of the toes and foot are largely controlled by the L5 nerve root so that compression of this root frequently causes discernible weakness. A large muscle like the quadriceps, on the other hand, is innervated by several roots so that involvement of only one of these roots is not so readily revealed. The extensors and flexors of the toes and ankles are

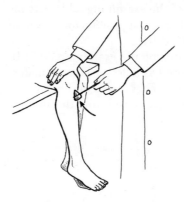

Figure 91.   The patellar reflex is best elicited when the patient's legs are hanging over the edge of the bed or examining table.

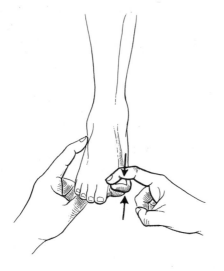

Figure 92.   Testing extension strength of the great toe. The tendon of the extensor hallucis longus can be seen; the finger is palpating the short extensors of the toes. In long-standing cases of nerve root compression, atrophy of the short toe extensors can be seen and palpated.

tested by asking the patient to move the toes and ankle against resistance and comparing both sides (Fig. 92).

Straight leg raising, or the Lasègue test, is carried out by slowly elevating the patient's leg without bending the knee. Normally it should be possible to raise the limb to a right angle with the table or a full 90 degrees. If pain is appreciated before this point is reached, the degree of elevation possible before pain is appreciated is noted and compared with the opposite side (Fig. 93). This test and all its many variants are based on the stretching of the sciatic nerve associated with straight leg raising. If any of the nerve roots that make up the sciatic nerve are compressed, stretching the main nerve trunk will aggravate symptoms from the already compromised nerve root by means of the reflected tug.

The Patrick test is carried out by flexing the thigh and knee, placing the external malleolus upon the opposite patella, and laterally depressing the knee (Fig. 94). This causes flexion, external rotation, and abduction of

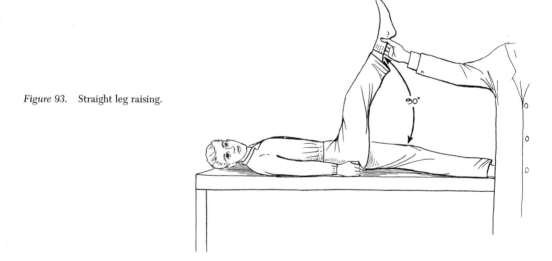

Figure 93. Straight leg raising.

90°

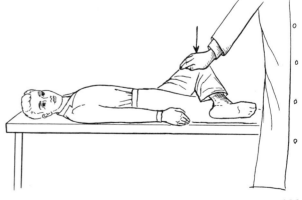

Figure 94. Patrick's test for involvement of the hip.

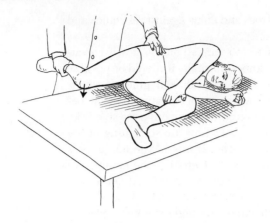

Figure 95. Ober's test for contraction of the tensor fasciae latae.

the hip joint; a positive test indicates a lesion of the hip joint, iliopsoas muscle spasm, or a sacroiliac lesion, as distinguished from a spinal lesion.

In performing the Ober test the patient is then placed on his side to determine whether contraction of the iliotibial band is present. The patient lies on his side with the side to be tested uppermost. The lower thigh and knee are flexed at a 90 degree angle; with the upper knee flexed at a right angle, the thigh is slowly extended until it is in line with the body. If the iliotibial band is contracted, the thigh will remain passively abducted, whereas the normal patient will allow the tested knee to drop to the examining table without difficulty (Fig. 95).

CHRONIC LUMBOSACRAL STRAIN

Chronic lumbosacral strain is the most common low back problem encountered in practice. It is a disease of middle age, and although it is not so painful as many of the other forms of low back pain, treatment of this condition is difficult and often falls short of the mark.

Symptoms and Signs

Most individuals complain of an aching discomfort in the lumbosacral region. The pain often covers a wide area rather than being confined to a specific spot and is rarely of great severity; it is usually described as "fairly severe" or even "mild." This discomfort has usually been present for a prolonged and not too definite time, and although a history of a fall or injury is often elicited, careful questioning usually reveals that the discomfort antedates the trauma. Aside from pain, the single most common denominator associated with this syndrome is fatigue. The patient often complains that the pain occurs during periods of general fatigue and may indicate that despite adequate hours of sleep, fatigue is constantly present. Frequently patients even complain of a "tired feeling" in the back instead of pain. Almost any activity can aggravate the pain and bed rest usually relieves it. The posture and general carriage are usually poor and the patient is often overweight. The musculature is often generally atonic and flabby.

Examination usually reveals fairly good mobility of the lumbar spine with no muscle spasm. The reflex and sensory examinations and straight leg raising tests are usually normal. X-rays of the spine may reveal increase of the normal lumbar curvature.

Pathophysiology

This syndrome results from deterioration of muscles and ligaments and may occur when because of ignorance or indolence patients treat their bodies as if they were inert shells designed only to house their digestive systems and requiring no special attention. This abuse and neglect is invariably associated with poor general hygiene. Constipation, poor diet, inadequate rest, and a host of other poor health habits are usually elicited in the history. A somewhat flat affect is often characteristic. To put it another way, I cannot recall seeing this syndrome in clear eyed, purposeful, aggressive individuals. The erect carriage involves a mental as well as physical state of health.

Women are more frequently affected by these symptoms and housewives are particularly susceptible. The fashionable high heels and girdles undoubtedly play some role in this syndrome. The routine wearing of high heels requires a compensatory adjustment of the spine to maintain the erect posture. This involves an increase of the lumbar curvature, which, in the presence of flabby musculature, creates a disproportionate strain upon the lower back. The wearing of a properly fitted corset or girdle could conceivably be of some benefit in lending support to the inadequate musculature. However, many housewives are accustomed to performing their duties about the house without wearing such a garment, reserving its use to occasions when they are "going out" and wish to create the impression of being trim and slim. I personally categorize girdles worn for fashion and high heeled shoes as one step removed from the ancient Chinese custom of binding women's feet.

Management

In dealing with a problem of this nature that has been present for a prolonged period of time a thorough work-up is essential. The physician must be certain that rectal or pelvic disease is not causing the patient's symptoms, and routine laboratory studies, in addition to x-rays of the lumbar and thoracic spine, must be obtained. A careful, painstaking study of this nature is the first important step in the management of the syndrome, since it gives a certain degree of confidence and trust to the patient in addition to being of great value to the physician in ruling out a variety of occult conditions that may be associated with backache. Complete confidence in the physician and a willingness to follow his instructions carefully are of prime importance, since the treatment involves many changes in the patient's mode

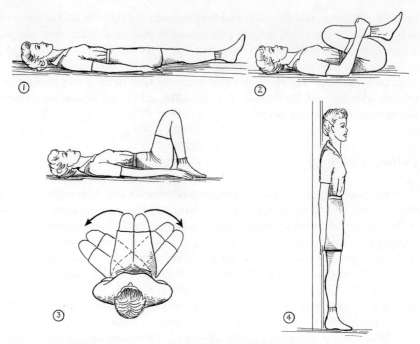

Figure 96. Low back exercises. (1) Lying on the back, flatten the lumbar region against the floor, maintaining the position for a count of three. Repeat three times. (2) Lying on the back, slowly pull the knees against the chest, clasp hands across the knees, and maintain this position for a count of three. Repeat three times. (3) Lying on the back, bring both knees up to a bent position, feet resting on the floor. Rotate the pelvis and legs to the right and then to the left side of body. Repeat once. (4) In the erect position, press back against a wall and contract the abdomen for a count of five. Repeat three times.

of living. A detailed explanation to the patient, using simple terms, is of great value in securing this confidence and cooperation. There are a variety of corrective postural exercises designed to increase the strength of the low back muscles. The following exercises do not require excessive exertion and can be performed in a short period of time (Fig. 96).

Exercise 1.   Lie on the back and flatten the lumbar region against the floor, maintaining the position for a count of three. Repeat three times.

Exercise 2.   Lie on the back and slowly pull the knees against the chest. Clasp hands across the knees and maintain this position for a count of three. Repeat three times.

Exercise 3.   Lie on the back and bring both knees up to a bent position with the feet resting on the floor. Rotate pelvis and legs to the right and then the left side of body. Repeat once.

Exercise 4.   In the erect position, press back against the wall and contract the abdomen for a count of five. Repeat three times.

If the patient is overweight, a gradual weight reduction program is started. A moderate decrease to a two-inch heel length, rather than a sudden shift to a low heel, is advisable in women accustomed to wearing extremely high heeled shoes. An abrupt reduction of heel length may aggravate symptoms by placing the shortened Achilles tendon on stretch.

Adequate rest should include eight hours of sleep at night supplemented by a one-hour period of bed rest in the afternoon. The mattress should be firm enough to support the reclining body without sagging in the lumbosacral region. A plywood board inserted between the spring and the mattress usually corrects a moderate sag. Many patients sleep on bed boards or even buy a special orthopedic mattress and then sit in overstuffed furniture during their waking hours. Firm, straight chairs support the back best, and if a great deal of driving is done, an auto seat back frame should be used. Several adequate varieties of these are available on the general market.

It usually requires several months before such a program is effective in eliminating symptoms, and it is usually necessary to utilize a canvas belt designed to support the low back and abdominal muscles. As muscle tone and strength increase, this belt can be discarded.

ACUTE LUMBOSACRAL STRAIN

This syndrome is brought on by injury to the lower back from lifting excessive loads or from other causes, including direct trauma to the back or falls in which the low back region is twisted.

Signs and Symptoms

The precipitating trauma to the low back region invariably causes immediate discomfort. In many cases the initial pain is not unduly severe but is appreciated mainly as a stiffness of the low back region, which is due largely to the secondary muscle spasm. The patient may continue to work or remain active in the hope that the activity will serve to "work out" the muscle spasm. Severe acute muscle spasm that has resulted from trauma frequently worsens with activity so that the patient may eventually become grossly incapacitated. It is not unusual to find the patient lying in bed or even on the floor suffering so severely that not only is he unable to move himself, but even the gentlest movement of the stretcher used to transport him to the hospital causes excruciating discomfort. Less often the initial pain is severe enough to cause such total disability.

The average acute lumbosacral strain is less severe and is manifested as low back discomfort, which is usually worse on one side, the most severe pain often being localized to a rather discrete area. Examination of the back reveals severe bilateral or unilateral spasm of the lumbar paraspinal muscles. Forward bending causes increased discomfort with limited mobility of the lumbar spine. If the paraspinal muscle spasm is unilateral, lateral bending of the body away from the side of spasm is painful, while the same movement toward the muscle spasm is less uncomfortable and in some cases actually relieves the pain. Occasionally, with unilateral muscle spasm, lumbar scoliosis

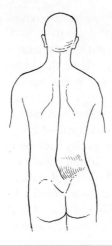

Figure 97. If paraspinal muscle spasm is unilateral, lumbar scoliosis may result with the concavity toward the side of the spasm.

is seen with the concavity toward the side of the spasm (Fig. 97). When the spasm is severe and widespread, any body movement including movement of the lower extremities may be painful. Reflex and sensory examinations are normal. The x-rays of the lumbosacral spine are often normal. They may, however, reveal some straightening of the normal lumbar curvature, and when the muscle spasm is unilateral, lumbar scoliosis may be noted.

Management

A patient who is so incapacitated with an acute lumbosacral strain that he is unable to work should be placed at bed rest. As in all low back problems, bed boards or a firm mattress is necessary. Muscle relaxants are helpful in reducing the muscle spasm, but it may be necessary to use narcotics in fairly substantial dosages if pain persists during bed rest. A natural reluctance to use narcotics in what may eventuate into a long, drawn out, chronic problem may impel the physician to prescribe small doses, which will be ineffective. Once the physician decides that narcotics are needed, one or two large doses are more effective in relaxing muscle spasm than several smaller doses.

Physiotherapy in the form of heat and possibly gentle massage is often helpful. If muscle spasm persists in spite of bed rest and medication, infiltration of the paraspinal muscle with a local anesthetic may offer prompt relief, which frequently lasts beyond the pharmacologic duration of the drug.

Unless an underlying condition, such as a herniated disc or a fracture, is present, the muscle spasm invariably improves with bed rest. With the subsidence of muscle spasm the patient will be comfortable as long as he remains in bed. Before ambulation, which may cause a prompt return of the muscle spasm, is permitted, several nonstrenuous low back exercises should be performed while lying in bed. The first three exercises described in the discussion on chronic low back strain are suitable. Exercises 1 and 2 are performed several times daily, and if no discomfort is appreciated exercise 3 is added. After several days of such mobilizing exercises the patient is ambulated wearing a Knight spinal brace for support of the lower back

(Fig. 98). This brace is worn for six weeks whenever the patient is out of bed for any activity, including resting in a chair. Activities are increased progressively until the patient can take up his normal endeavors. During the period of convalescence, the patient should be supervised carefully. Excessive exercise may cause exacerbation of the muscle spasm, while excessive rest may not only prolong the recovery period but create a so-called "low back neurosis" in which the patient considers himself an invalid; in fact, he may eventually develop into an invalid if not carefully handled.

Manipulative therapy to the lower back is often effective in the treatment of the residuals of an acute low back strain. The improvement resulting from manipulation is chiefly due to stretching of muscles and tendons that have become contracted and shortened as a result of spasm. In addition, the fibrous tissues surrounding the joints of the back may become contracted and even develop adhesions after prolonged immobility of the lower back. Manipulation may be helpful in stretching these adherent tissues.

There is no basis to the nonmedical claims that manipulation produces an "adjustment" or realignment of subluxated vertebrae. This is one of the oldest forms of therapy, having been employed by Hippocrates and followed by a distinguished list of physicians. As this form of treatment was preempted by nonmedical practitioners, medical doctors tended to dissociate themselves completely, ignoring any possible merits of the treatment. Let me emphasize that any "magic" resulting from the "laying on of hands" occurs only in functional or hysterical cases, but it is certainly a helpful adjuvant when used in conjunction with the other forms of available therapy.

One of the disadvantages of this form of therapy is the practice necessary to acquire some skill in its use. It is as much of a skill as surgery, and although no untrained physician would expect to perform competent neurosurgery after reading a brief description of a brain operation, many doctors attempt to manipulate a back with little or no instruction. After a few such unsuccessful attempts they may then condemn manipulation as being of no value. Before attempting a series of manipulative procedures on a patient with low back pain, the manipulator should practice on a normal subject

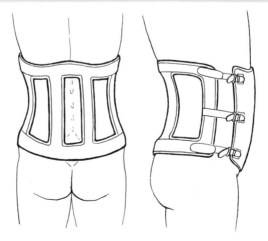

Figure 98.   Knight spinal brace.

so that he will be completely familiar with the normal resistance and mobility of each maneuver. No properly performed manipulation should cause discomfort to the normal subject, and the session should not be a painful one to the patient. If a particular maneuver causes discomfort, it is preferable to perform it gently short of pain and to repeat it at a subsequent session.

Herniated discs, possible spinal tumors, vertebral fractures, and dislocations are all contraindications to manipulation. Manipulation under anesthesia provides muscle relaxation in those individuals with such severe muscle spasm that the movements would not be tolerated, but it is also dangerous, since the degree of relaxation may be so great as to allow injury to the spine from hypermanipulation. I am opposed to the use of anesthesia by any but

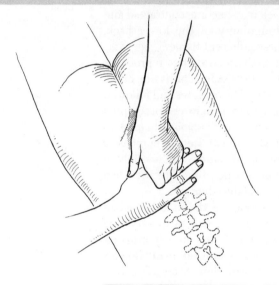

Figure 99. Spinal thrust. The palm of the right hand is placed on the back, perpendicular to the spinal axis with the spinous processes just proximal to the fifth metacarpophalangeal joint. Using the left hand for reenforcement, make a short rapid thrust, starting at the lumbosacral joint and progressing along each interspace to the midthoracic spine. The direction of the thrust is downward and toward the head.

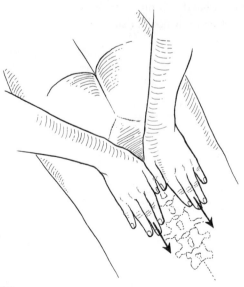

Figure 100. Paraspinal thrust. The hands are placed on either side of the spinous processes with the fingers pointed toward the patient's head. Starting in the lumbosacral region, make a series of short rapid thrusts, using the heels of the hands, at each interspace up to the midthoracic spine. The direction of force is downward and toward the head.

the most experienced operator and believe that with bed rest, medication, and patience the most severe muscle spasm can eventually be controlled to a degree at which manipulation may be tolerated.

Maneuver 1 (Spinal Thrust).   With the patient lying on an examining table in the prone position, the physician stands on the patient's right side facing the patient (Fig. 99). The palm of the right hand is placed on the back perpendicular to the spinal axis with the spinous processes just proximal to the fifth metacarpophalangeal joint. Using the left hand for reenforcement, one makes a short rapid thrust, starting at the lumbosacral joint and progressing along each interspace to the midthoracic spine. The direction of the thrust is downward and toward the head.

Maneuver 2 (Paraspinal Thrust).   With the patient and the therapist in the same position as for maneuver 1, the physician's hands are placed on either side of the spinous processes with the fingers pointed toward the patient's head. Starting in the lumbosacral region, the physician makes a series of short rapid thrusts, using the palms of the hands, at each interval up to the midthoracic spine (Fig. 100). As in the spinal thrust, the direction of force is downward and toward the head.

Maneuver 3 (Hyperextension of the Thigh).   With the patient in the prone position, the manipulator places his left hand over the right buttock, exerting a steady, firm, downward pressure (Fig. 101). With the knee in extension the right thigh is hyperextended. This maneuver is repeated on the opposite side.

Maneuver 4 (Spinal Hyperextension and Pelvic Rotation).   With the patient in prone position, the manipulator stands at the foot of the table (Fig. 102). While the patient maintains the lower extremities in extension, the physician grasps both feet and elevates the extremities in wheelbarrow fashion causing hyperextension of the spine. Maintaining one extremity elevated, the physician lowers the other to the table; the same maneuver is repeated with the opposite leg.

Maneuver 5 (Backward and Forward Spinal Torsion).   The patient is placed on his left side with the left lower extremity extended and the

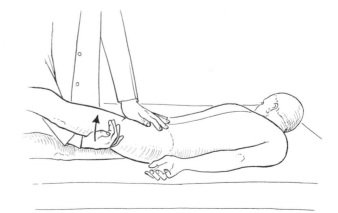

Figure 101. Hyperextension of the thigh. With the left hand exerting a steady, firm, downward pressure upon the right buttock, the left thigh is hyperextended with the knee in extension. This maneuver is repeated on the opposite side.

139

right hip and knee flexed (Fig. 103). The patient's right hand is placed over his right breast. Standing behind the patient, the physician places his right hand over the right iliac crest and his left hand upon the right shoulder. A forward torsion movement is then performed by simultaneously drawing the right shoulder backward and exerting a sudden forward and downward thrust on the right ilium. This movement, which is often associated with a snapping sound, produces stretching of the right posterior sacroiliac ligament and the right iliolumbar ligament as well as rotation of the interlaminar joints of the lumbar and lower thoracic vertebrae.

The manipulator then performs a backward torsion movement by thrusting the shoulder forward and drawing the right ilium backward. This stretches the right anterior sacroiliac ligament and rotates the vertebral inter-laminar joints in the opposite direction. The same maneuver is repeated with the patient on his right side.

Maneuver 6 (Passive Straight Leg Raising). With the patient in a supine position, the lower extremity is slowly elevated with the knee extended

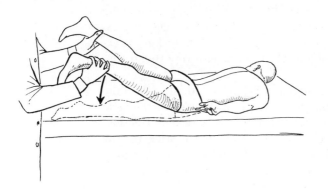

Figure 102. Spinal hyperextension and pelvic rotation. While the patient maintains the lower extremities in extension, grasp both feet and elevate the extremities in wheelbarrow fashion, causing hyperextension of the spine. Maintaining one extremity elevated, lower the other to the table. Repeat the same maneuver with the opposite leg.

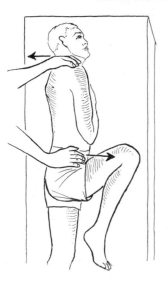

Figure 103. Backward and forward spinal torsion. The patient is placed on his left side with the left lower extremity extended and the right hip and knee flexed. The patient's right hand is placed over his right breast. Standing behind the patient, the physician places his right hand over the right iliac crest and his left hand upon the right shoulder. A forward torsion movement is then performed by simultaneously drawing the right shoulder backward and exerting a sudden forward and downward thrust of the right ilium. A backward torsion movement is then carried out by thrusting the shoulder forward and drawing the ilium backward. The maneuver is repeated with the patient on his right side.

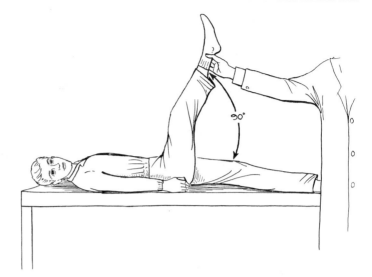

Figure 104. Passive straight leg raising. The lower extremity is elevated slowly with the knee extended. This maneuver is performed short of producing pain or to an angulation of 90°.

(Fig. 104). This maneuver is performed short of producing pain or to an angulation of 90 degrees. The maneuver is repeated with the opposite leg.

The patient should experience definite improvement of symptoms following the manipulative session. If no relief occurs after a properly performed manipulation, the underlying disease will not respond to this treatment and there is no need for a repeat session. Prompt ambulation following manipulation is the rule. Muscle reeducation by means of postural exercises may be helpful when used in conjunction with this treatment.

THE HERNIATED LUMBAR DISC

Physicians as a group lean toward the conservative side and are not overly quick to accept a new concept. However, once the principle has become established, several years elapse before it ceases to be overemphasized and assumes its deserved position. The lumbar disc concept is probably now reaching its proper level and the number of laminectomies performed is diminishing.

Pathophysiology

If all the intervertebral discs were removed, the unfortunate individual subjected to this procedure would be 20 to 25 per cent shorter. Careful measurements taken in the morning and repeated in the evening on several hundred people have demonstrated a decrease in height at the end of the day, which is presumably due to loss of some of the water content of the intervertebral discs coincident with weight bearing.

Because of their position in the lordotic curve of the lumbar spine, the discs between the fourth and fifth lumbar vertebrae and the fifth lumbar and

141

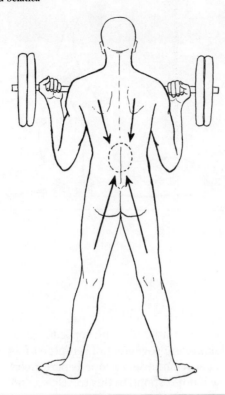

Figure 105. The stress of weight-bearing upon the low back.

first sacral vertebrae are subjected to the greatest weight bearing stress and are most severely compressed posteriorly (Fig. 105). This stress may cause degenerative changes in the somewhat elastic ring of the annulus fibrosus, which normally confines the soft, gelatinous remnant of the embryonic notochord, the nucleus pulposus. Once degenerative changes occur, healing rarely occurs because of the constant weight bearing and the relatively poor blood supply to the intervertebral disc. The annulus fibrosus is weaker posteriorly so that degeneration of this structure would be likely to allow posterior protrusions of the nucleus pulposus. This in turn produces an abnormal pressure upon the posterior spinal ligament, which is thick in the center and fairly thin laterally. It is the thick central portion of the posterior spinal ligament that causes most intervertebral discs to protrude laterally.

Signs and Symptoms

Low back pain associated with sciatica, the classic picture of lumbar disc disease, is usually preceded by a prolonged period of intermittent, mild low back pain. This pain is often so insidious in onset that patients in many cases are unable to recall its duration. Such statements as "I have always had a weak back" are common. Mild low back discomfort results from a variety of activities and subsides spontaneously with rest. The patient may never consult a physician because of low back pains until an episode occurs that is severe enough to cause incapacitation and does not subside spontaneously. Frequently a specific episode is cited by the patient as the precipitating cause of the attack. This may be a trauma, such as lifting a heavy weight and appreciating "a sudden snap in my back" or a fall, or may even result when the patient bends forward to pick up a piece of paper or other object of negligible weight. Severe intractable low back pain eventually is associated with sciatica.

At this point in the clinical course the pain has two distinct components, the low back pain described as aching and the sciatica variously described as electric shock-like, pins and needles sensation, numbness, or stabbing pains. The pain is aggravated by any activity that involves weight bearing and stress upon the lumbar area, including standing, walking, and prolonged driving. Coughing, sneezing, and straining at stool cause a sudden increase in the pain. Improvement, if not complete relief of pain, invariably results from lying down.

The symptoms just described occur when the most commonly seen "laterally protruded disc" produces the "single root syndrome." This refers to compression of one nerve root just before it passes out of the spine through the intervertebral foramen (Figs. 106, 107). The so-called "midline disc protrusion" may be marked by pain involving only the lower back, or if the lesion is sufficiently large, the pain may radiate down both lower extremities. An uncommon but dangerous form of lumbar disc disease is the sudden massive extrusion that creates extensive compression of the cauda equina and, in addition to pain, causes sphincter paralysis and paraplegia.

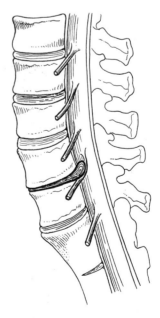

Figure 106.   Herniated L4–5 disc causing nerve root compression.

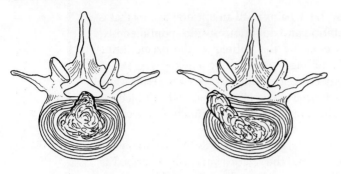

Figure 107. Central and lateral disc herniations.

Examination

Paraspinal muscle spasm with impaired mobility of the lumbar spine on forward bending and pain on straight leg raising can be considered general signs of lumbar disc disease. The majority of lumbar disc syndromes occur between the fourth and fifth lumbar vertebrae (or L4-L5) and the fifth lumbar and first sacral vertebrae (or L5-S1), and several specific signs, if present, indicate the interspace involved.

The L5-S1 disc protrusion involves the first sacral nerve root. A diminished or absent Achilles reflex and numbness along the lateral aspect of the foot point to involvement of the first sacral nerve root. Occasionally, when the painful sciatic radiation is appreciated in the foot, the patient states that the pain extends only into the lateral aspect of the foot (Fig. 108).

The L4-L5 disc protrusion, which involves the fifth lumbar nerve root,

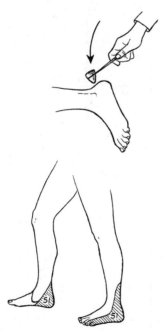

Figure 108. Characteristic of L5–S1 disc herniation are the diminished or absent Achilles reflex and numbness within the S1 nerve root dermatome.

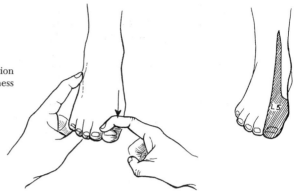

Figure 109.   Characteristic of L4–L5 disc herniation are weakness of great toe extension and numbness within the L5 nerve root dermatome.

produces no change in the Achilles reflex; a faint zone of hypesthesia may be elicited over the dorsum of the foot, extending into the great toe, within the L5 nerve root dermatome. Fifth lumbar nerve root involvement is likely to cause some extensor motor weakness, which can be elicited by careful examination of the extensors of the great toe (Fig. 109).

Management

The patient with an acute attack of lumbar disc disease should be hospitalized if a trial of bed rest at home for one week is not adequate to alleviate the symptoms. In the hospital, absolute bed rest on a firm mattress is a standard order for every patient admitted with lumbar disc disease. Muscle relaxants may be helpful in relieving the discomfort of paraspinal muscle spasm. The patient should be maintained as pain-free as possible with the use of analgesics. Frequently aspirin may be adequate, but codeine, Demerol, or morphine may be required, particularly during the first 24 to 48 hours, when the symptoms may be acute. The possible constipating action of the opiates must be kept in mind; a nightly laxative, such as milk of magnesia, helps eliminate this complication, since straining at stool is to be avoided. The use of heat over the painful region may be helpful in relieving muscle spasm, but we do not routinely employ massage or exercise in any form during the acute phase.

The benefits to be derived from the use of traction in lumbar disc disease are open to question. Some physicians believe that the symptomatic improvement attributed to traction is actually due to bed rest, nothing being contributed by the traction. Although we are inclined to agree with this view from an academic standpoint, we routinely employ traction with bed rest in almost every lumbar disc problem. This technique imparts to the patient a feeling of receiving constant treatment, while if he is confined to bed without traction, he frequently voices the complaint, "Nothing is being done for me." We prefer the so-called "pelvic traction," which employs a snug canvas girdle encircling the pelvis and hips with traction straps leading from this girdle to weights hung at the foot of the bed (Fig. 110). Fifteen to 30 pounds of weight can be utilized, and the foot of the bed should be slightly elevated so that the weight of the patient's body may provide countertraction and he will not be constantly pulled toward the foot of the bed. Leg traction, or Buck's extension, which employs the pull directly upon the lower extremities, should never be used for disc disease (Fig. 111).

Although the merits of pelvic traction are equivocal, it is contrary to all reasonable expectation for leg traction, which must transmit a force through the knee and hip joints before involving the intervertebral joints, to be effective. In addition, this type of traction prevents movement of the lower extremities, which in the case of prolonged bed rest may lead to occasional venous stasis complications, such as phlebothrombosis. The patient in pelvic traction can move his lower extremities freely, and this is helpful in preventing such complications.

The patient is maintained at bed rest with traction until all pain has subsided; only then should mobilization be permitted. Before permitting the patient to ambulate, he should be fitted with a Knight spinal brace, which serves to splint the lumbar spine. Mobilization should be carried out in graduated stages, and strict avoidance of forward bending, heavy lifting, and climbing stairs is recommended for the first two weeks. The brace is worn for at least eight weeks after which it can be slowly discarded for progressively increasing periods of time.

Only after an adequate trial of conservative management has failed should surgery be considered.

It should be emphasized that patients who present marked motor weakness, such as foot drop, or evidence of extensive compression of the cauda equina with motor involvement of both lower extremities and sphincter

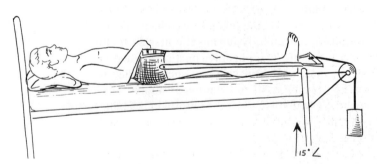

Figure 110. Pelvic traction. Elevation of foot of bed allows weight of the patient's body to provide countertraction.

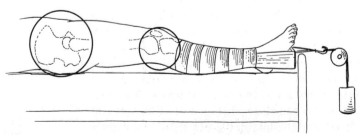

Figure 111. Buck's extension is a mechanically inefficient method of traction for low back pain, since the traction force must be transmitted through the knee and hip joints before affecting the low back.

palsy are to be considered surgical emergencies. Treating such individuals conservatively is not only poor management but can lead to irreversible neurologic damage.

Myelography should never be used routinely as a diagnostic aid to confirm the presence of a protruded disc. This study is reserved for those patients who have had an adequate trial of conservative treatment without relief of symptoms and are to be considered for surgery.

Twenty years ago Lipiodol was the only available radiopaque material for myelograms, and because of its extremely high viscosity some difficulty was encountered in obtaining the desired free flow within the subarachnoid space, in addition to the problem of removing this molasses-like substance after completion of the myelogram. It was common practice in many clinics to leave this contrast material within the subarachnoid space, resulting in adhesive arachnoiditis in a considerable number of patients. The present use of Pantopaque, which is far less irritating and which can be easily removed since it is less viscous, has made myelography a relatively innocuous procedure.

The test involves the introduction of Pantopaque into the subarachnoid space through a lumbar puncture needle. By means of a tilt table with the patient in prone position, the Pantopaque is moved under fluoroscopic control up and down the portion of the spine to be studied, and films are obtained when the Pantopaque is pooled within selected segments of the spine. Any extensive mass capable of causing pressure upon the nerve roots displaces the opaque column and is referred to as a filling defect. After satisfactory films are obtained, the Pantopaque is removed through the original lumbar puncture needle, which has been maintained in place, until all the Pantopaque is aspirated and the procedure is completed.

The occasional mishap occurring with this test is often related to the lumbar puncture technique employed. The use of any needle other than an 18-gauge lumbar puncture needle is ill advised, since complete removal of the oily opaque material is difficult with a finer needle. Oblique introduction of the needle causes the needle point to lodge against the lateral portion of the subarachnoid space. This position may offer no problem when the Pantopaque is introduced, but upon attempted withdrawal of the substance, a nerve root may be drawn up into the aspirating lumen of the needle, causing severe discomfort and preventing complete removal of the Pantopaque.

Introduction of the Pantopaque into the subdural rather than the subarachnoid space is not only painful but is worthless from a diagnostic standpoint. This error is made when the bevel of the needle is only partly within the subarachnoid space and the arachnoid membrane is "tented" upon the needle point rather than being completely perforated by the needle. The "jet stream" of the Pantopaque, as it is introduced through the lumen of the needle, may push the arachnoid membrane completely off the needle point, and the oil collects within this false subdural space between the dura and the arachnoid (Fig. 112).

Most of these errors can be avoided by performing the lumbar puncture with the patient in the sitting rather than in the usual lateral recumbent position. Central placement of the needle is facilitated by avoiding the error

147

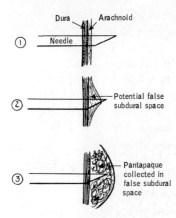

Dura   Arachnoid

① ── Needle

② ──── Potential false
         subdural space

③ ──── Pantapaque
         collected in
         false subdural
         space

Figure 112. If the lumbar puncture needle is poorly placed when injecting Pantopaque for a myelogram, the Pantopaque may be injected into the subdural space resulting in a worthless study. (1) Well-positioned needle has perforated both the dura and the arachnoid. (2) Poorly positioned lumbar puncture needle with the bevel through the dura but not completely through the thin filmy arachnoid. (3) Pantopaque injected through needle, illustrated in (2), may cause the filmy arachnoid membrane to be pushed forward by the force of the injected material, creating a false space between the dura and the arachnoid (subdural space) within which the pantopaque is deposited.

attendant upon lateral sag of soft tissues over the spine when the patient is in the lateral position. The subdural injection is also avoided by "tapping" the sitting patient, since in the erect position the tall subarachnoid column develops increased hydrostatic pressure and distention within the caudal sac. Thus, the arachnoid membrane is pressed against the point of the needle, making complete perforation more certain.

Surgery

Removal of a herniated lumbar disc is not a particularly formidable procedure when performed by an experienced surgeon. By means of a subperiosteal muscle dissection, the spines and lamina of the appropriate interspace are exposed. The space between the lamina is enlarged by removing the overhanging edge of the superior lamina. Upon medial retraction of the nerve root, the protruded disc is exposed. The posterior longitudinal ligament is incised and the disc is removed, using a pituitary forceps to empty the disc space as completely as possible of all fragments of disc material. Following the disc removal, the nerve root, which is usually swollen, is decompressed within its intervertebral foramen by performing a foraminotomy or an unroofing of the dorsal portion of this bony canal (Fig. 113). The patient is ambulated on the day following surgery and discharged from the hospital approximately a week after surgery. A minimum of six weeks' convalescence is required before allowing desk workers to return to employment and ten to twelve weeks for manual workers. The patient is fitted with a Knight spinal brace following lumbar disc surgery, and this appliance is worn for six weeks whenever he is out of bed.

Spinal fusion is rarely performed, in our practice, as a combined procedure following the disc removal. Since the majority of patients do very well after removal of the disc alone, the greatly increased convalescence required following a fusion procedure would be an unnecessary period of inactivity and discomfort borne by the patient. Less than 3 per cent of patients with ruptured discs require fusion, and this can be performed as a

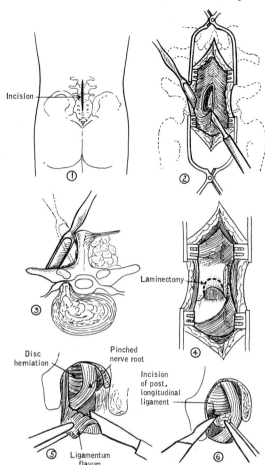

Figure 113. Lumbar disc surgery. (1) Incision. (2 & 3) Subperiosteal muscle dissection. (4) The interspace is enlarged by rongeuring the overhanging edge of the superior lamina. (5) Excising the yellow ligament to expose the nerve root compresed by a herniated disc. (6) Piecemeal removal of herniated disc.

separate procedure. When properly managed, 90 per cent of patients having surgery for herniated lumbar discs make a good recovery.

LOW BACK PAIN ASSOCIATED WITH OSTEOPOROSIS

Osteoporosis is a metabolic bone disease commonly found in the elderly female. One should remember that it can occur at all ages and in both sexes. In addition to its occurrence as a specific pathologic entity, it may also occur in association with several systemic diseases.

Pathophysiology

The deficiency of bone substance may develop from absorption of bone matrix with poor replacement, from destruction of bone matrix, or from inadequate production of matrix. The factors vital to formation of bone matrix

149

are estrogens, androgens, vitamin C, and adequate protein intake. Any disease or condition influencing one or several of these factors will produce osteoporosis.

Symptoms and Signs

Osteoporosis may exist for years without causing any symptoms until trauma causes collapse of one or more vertebral bodies. This trauma may be quite minor, such as stepping down from a high curb or picking up a relatively light object. In some cases, no specific trauma can be recalled. Generalized low back pain of an aching nature is usually associated with localized tenderness over the collapsed vertebra. Tenderness over all the long bones, particularly those near the surface of the skin, such as the tibia or the ulna, is noted when the condition is generalized.

Diagnosis

The senile patient with persistent low back pain should always be considered an osteoporosis suspect. X-ray of the spine may reveal vertebral collapse and radiolucency of the skeleton as a whole. Laboratory studies, including serum calcium, phosphorus, and alkaline phosphatase, are usually within normal limits.

Secondary osteoporosis should be suspected in patients with Cushing's syndrome, acromegaly, scurvy, and thyrotoxicosis who complain of low back pain.

Treatment

An adequate intake of vitamins C and D, calcium, and phosphorus must be assured. A high protein diet is important since the general nutritional state is often inadequate. To stimulate production of bone matrix, androgens and estrogens are administered simultaneously.

A common error in the management of this problem is to allow the patient to remain immobilized in bed for prolonged periods. Increased activity is of value in producing deposition of calcium in the affected bone by allowing the osteoblasts to receive the necessary stimuli. Any means of encouraging early activity in these elderly uncomfortable patients should be utilized, including analgesics, physiotherapy, and a low back support to reduce discomfort during ambulation.

LOW BACK PAIN AND CONGENITAL ANOMALIES

A number of congenital variations in the anatomy of the lumbar spine are often revealed by x-ray films. These anomalies are generally incidental findings, since the usual reason for obtaining these x-ray films is an acute problem, such as strain or trauma. Such abnormalities as lumbarized sacral vertebrae, sacralized lumbar vertebrae, spina bifida, hemivertebrae, or enlarged transverse processes rarely produce symptoms. The two anomalies that may cause difficulty are spondylolisthesis and scoliosis.

Spondylolisthesis

Spondylolisthesis literally translated means slipping of a vertebra. It is characterized by a defect in the neural arch with a fibrous pseudoarthrosis present at the junction of the neural arch and the vertebral body in place of the normal bony union. The failure of fusion between the vertebral body and pedicle is congenital, but the subsequent vertebral displacement is related to superimposed trauma. The lesion occurs most commonly in the fifth and less commonly in the fourth lumbar vertebrae. If this weakened area is subjected to stress, forward displacement of one vertebra upon the other may occur (Fig. 114). If the defect is present only unilaterally, or is present bilaterally without anterior displacement, the condition is termed spondylolysis. Trauma may aggravate this condition, but it is unusual for a patient who has never experienced low back symptoms to be incapacitated by a single injury.

Signs and Symptoms. Usually the gradual onset of symptoms occurs within the late twenties and early thirties. The initial symptom is usually generalized aching discomfort in the low back region. With progressive anterior slipping of the affected vertebra, foraminal impingement upon the nerve root occurs, and this may be heralded by extension of the dull, dragging ache into one or both buttocks. As the nerve root compression worsens, sciatica may develop. This is likely to be unilateral but may be bilateral. The change in vertebral alignment may be associated with protrusion or even rupture of the intervertebral disc, which has a tendency to occur at the level immediately above the pedicle defect. The low back pain and sciatica are indistinguishable from the picture presented by the protruded lumbar disc.

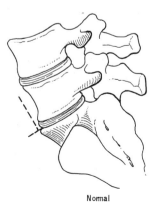

Figure 114. Ullman's line is extended upward at a right angle from the anterior edge of the first sacral vertebra to the superior surface of the sacrum. In cases of spondylolisthesis this line passes through the last lumbar vertebra.

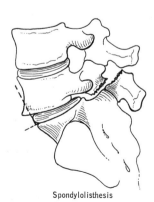

Normal

Spondylolisthesis

151

Management. The conservative treatment of this problem is similar to that used for the herniated disc, which includes bed rest and pelvic traction for the acute phase. After the patient is comfortable in bed, low back exercises are initiated and the patient is ambulated wearing a Knight spinal brace.

If this treatment is ineffective, surgical fusion with bone grafts to the area is indicated. Prior to any proposed surgery for spondylolisthesis, a myelogram should be performed to rule out the possibility of a herniated disc. If a herniated disc is present, it should be removed prior to fusion. In the event that sciatica is present without a herniated disc, the nerve root should be thoroughly decompressed by an extensive foraminotomy at the involved level prior to fusion.

Scoliosis

Congenital scoliosis is almost invariably related to anomalies of one or more vertebrae. Muscular and ligamentous contractures, the primary cause of congenital scoliosis, which produces secondary accomodative vertebral wedging, may occur but are extremely rare. It is not at all unusual to see scoliosis occurring as a complication of poliomyelitis, cerebral palsy, muscular dystrophy, and various diseases of the spine and thorax.

Whatever the etiology of scoliosis, it is usually asymptomatic unless the curve is extremely acute. Occasionally the progressive effect of the unequal stress upon the muscles of the back causes generalized muscle strain and aching. As a rule this problem is best managed conservatively with the wearing of a back support and postural exercise. Fusion is rarely necessary in the adult, but when a rapid increase in the curvature occurs in the child or teenager, surgery is most often indicated.

OSTEOARTHRITIS

Hypertrophic changes are often discovered as incidental findings on x-ray films obtained in cases of acute trauma. Extensive spurring at the anterior margin of the vertebral bodies and degenerative changes in the posterior articulations of the spine can be considered normal changes due to age or accumulated trauma over the years. Advanced hypertrophic changes in the spine may cause surprisingly little pain. When symptoms do occur, they are usually stiffness and a generalized mild ache, which is most marked upon arising in the morning, improves with activity during the day, and worsens again at night. Because of loss of normal mobility, an acute trauma or strain may cause more severe symptoms than would be experienced if these changes were not present.

Occasionally the intervertebral foramina may be encroached upon by spur formation of the apophyseal joints with subsequent nerve root pressure. The nerve root may also be impinged upon by hypertrophic lipping of the adjacent borders of two vertebrae projecting posteriorly in a fashion anatomically similar to a protruded disc (Fig. 115).

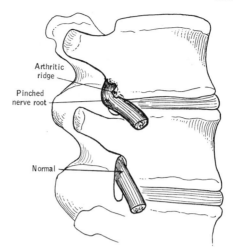

Figure 115. Osteoarthritic ridges producing nerve root compression.

Arthritic ridge

Pinched nerve root

Normal

Management of these problems consists of bed rest, pelvic traction, and physiotherapy. Low back support during ambulation by means of a brace is helpful.

When the nerve root pressure and sciatica do not subside with prolonged conservative management, decompression by means of a foraminotomy may be indicated. In our experience, this procedure is rarely necessary.

MERALGIA PARAESTHETICA

Neuralgia of the lateral femoral cutaneous nerve causes burning pain and numbness in the anterolateral aspect of the thigh, which may be confused with sciatica (Fig. 116).

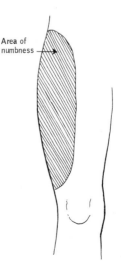

Area of numbness

Figure 116. Area affected by neuralgia of the lateral femoral cutaneous nerve.

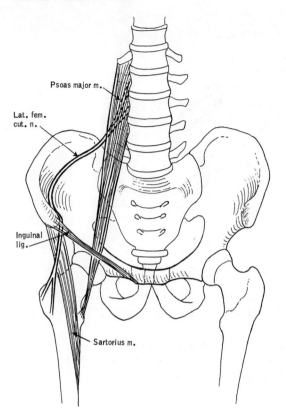

Psoas major m.

Lat. fem.
cut. n.

Inguinal
lig.

Sartorius m.

Figure 117. Common sites of compression
of lateral femoral cutaneous nerve.

Pathophysiology

Pressure on the lateral femoral cutaneous nerve at any point along its long
course may produce the syndrome. The nerve arises from the second and
third lumbar nerve roots, and hypertrophic arthritis of the upper lumbar
spine may cause nerve root compression. The nerve emerges at the lateral
border of the psoas muscle and can be involved at this site by a psoas abscess.
The nerve then runs across the iliacus muscle in the pelvis just beneath the
iliac fascia. Because of the superficial position in its long course within the
pelvis, it is quite vulnerable to pressure produced by intrapelvic lesions.
These include pregnancy, tumors, and infections. A traction neuritis of the
nerve may occur as it passes over the brim of the iliac crest and emerges from
the fascia under Poupart's ligament just medial to its attachment to the
anterior superior spine of the ilium. At this site, the nerve may be angulated
and stretched as the patient stands or walks. Individuals who have gained
weight and develop pendulous abdomens are particularly susceptible to
involvement at this site (Fig. 117). Braces, corsets, and trusses may cause
compression in this region. We once treated a dentist for this problem who
was accustomed to standing for long periods with his right anterior iliac
spine compressed against the arm of the dental chair.

Signs and Symptoms

The pain of meralgia paraesthetica involves the anterolateral thigh, and such adjectives as burning, glowing, tingling, and pins and needles are frequently elicited in the patient's description of the pain. The onset is usually spontaneous, but occasionally the patient may relate the development of pain to an unusually long walk or a prolonged period of standing. Symptoms are usually unilateral although rarely both thighs may be involved. The pain is usually decreased by lying down or sitting and is aggravated by walking about or prolonged standing. Although firm pressure upon the affected area may not be uncomfortable, light stroking of the skin may provoke an unpleasant tingling sensation. Men often complain that the fabric of their trousers brushes their thighs when they walk and causes this unpleasant dysesthesia.

Diagnosis

Although little difficulty is encountered in diagnosing this rather distinct clinical entity, determining the nature and site of the causative factor may be a problem. If the nerve is involved as it passes over the brim of the iliac crest, an analgesic block of the lateral femoral cutaneous nerve will relieve the pain (see Fig. 118). This block will be ineffective if the lesion is located proximally. In such instances, a complete neurologic survey, including x-rays of the lumbar spine, should be carried out. When the lesion is within the spine and is due to compression of the nerve roots by osteoarthritis or a herniated disc in the upper lumbar region, diminution of the patellar reflex and weakness and atrophy of the quadriceps muscle may be evident. Rectal and vaginal examination should be done, and in some cases, myelography may be necessary.

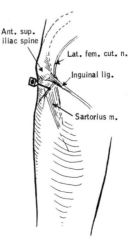

Figure 118. Injection of lateral femoral cutaneous nerve.

155

Treatment

If the lesion is located at the anterior superior iliac spine and is confirmed by subsidence of pain after analgesic block, repeated injections may create progressively longer pain-free intervals. If, after three blocks, no significant improvement is noted, they are not likely to be of therapeutic value.

The technique of blocking the lateral femoral cutaneous nerve in the thigh is simple. A 25-gauge, one-inch hypodermic needle is inserted at a site one-half inch medial and one inch below the anterior superior iliac spine. This is carefully advanced through the skin until paresthesias occur from contact with the nerve, at which point 10 cc. of Xylocaine is infiltrated. There is a tendency to insert the needle too deep, and this causes the anesthetic to be injected into the sartorius muscle and results in an ineffective block (Fig. 118).

The patient should be placed on a diet that will cause loss of excessive fat. Constricting straps around the abdomen must be eliminated. Women must discard tight corsets or girdles; men must substitute suspenders for belts.

At one time, section of the lateral femoral cutaneous nerve or neurolysis and transposition into a slot in the ilium was the treatment of choice. These procedures have not withstood the tests of time particularly well. When the nerve is sectioned, the pain may return because of the formation of a painful neuroma, which may also occur with transposition of the nerve. Spontaneous subsidence of the pain is likely to occur if a conservative regimen as that just outlined is carried out. When the syndrome is caused by a central lesion of the nerve or its spinal roots, proper therapy is directed appropriately.

chapter seven

Visceral Pain of the
Chest and Abdomen

chapter seven —

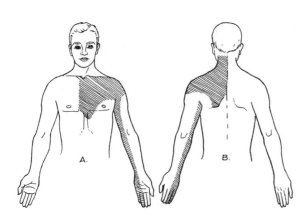

Figure 119. (A) The usual distribution of anginal pain. (B) Radiation of anginal pain into the left scapular region.

Visceral Pain of the
Chest and Abdomen

Most of the entities discussed in this section are not primarily pain problems, since general medical management of the disease usually produces both relief of pain and improved visceral function. In some cases, however, the standard methods of treatment are not effective in alleviating pain. This intractable discomfort may not only distress the patient but may be a detrimental factor in the general outcome of the illness. It is in these instances that various special pain relieving procedures may be considered.

CHEST PAIN

Cardiac Pain

Cardiac pain is the result of an inadequate supply of blood to the myocardium. When the patient is at rest the blood supply to the heart may be adequate, but when the work of the heart is increased there may be an insufficient supply of blood to meet the cardiac requirements. The coronary arteries, which supply the myocardium, may by partial or complete occlusion be responsible for insufficiency. An alteration in the quality of the circulating blood, as occurs in asphyxia, may also produce myocardial insufficiency. This imbalance between supply and demand produces myocardial ischemia, which is manifested clinically by pain or discomfort.

The term *angina pectoris* was introduced by William Heberden in 1768, when he described the syndrome of paroxysmal precordial or substernal pain frequently radiating to the shoulders and inner aspects of the arms. The literal meaning of angina is strangling, and the term refers to the characteristic respiratory oppression that is associated with the syndrome.

This syndrome can be precipitated by factors that transiently increase the work of the heart, such as physical exertion, a large meal, or emotional stress. Factors that cause a diminution in coronary flow may also be responsible for anginal pain. These include a fall in blood pressure from any cause, reflex vasomotor effects upon the coronary arteries from exposure to cold, emotional stress, or drugs, such as epinephrine. However, the most frequent cause of an inadequate coronary blood supply is arteriosclerosis.

Cardiac Pain Pathways. William Harvey, in the early 17th century, made the first recorded observation regarding cardiac sensitivity when this celebrated English physician was requested by King Charles I to examine the son of Count Montgomery. Young Viscount Montgomery had sustained a severe chest injury a few years before, which resulted in a large defect in the thoracic cavity. The wound healed with the heart exposed, and the child wore a shield over his chest to protect this organ. Harvey removed this cardiac cuirass and observed the beating heart. He thereupon stimulated the heart by touching, pinching, and pricking it. He noted that "unless when we touched the outer skin, or when he saw our fingers in the cavity, this young gentleman knew not that we touched the heart." He concluded that the heart was devoid of pain sensation. The error in his interpretation was due of course to failure to utilize an adequate physiologic stimulus. The adequate stimulus to the heart is myocardial anoxia, which acts on sensory nerve endings in the adventitia of the coronary arteries, in the subepicardial tissues, and in the myocardium.

These sensory axons pass through the superficial and deep cardiac plexuses and are relayed through the middle and inferior cervical sympathetic cardiac nerves and the upper thoracic sympathetic cardiac nerves to reach the upper four thoracic paravertebral sympathetic ganglia. The sensory fibers pass through the ganglia and their corresponding white rami communicantes without interruption to the upper four thoracic posterior spinal roots to reach the spinal cord. Within the cord the fibers synapse to enter the spinothalamic tract, which transmits the pain impulses to the brain (Fig. 120). An understanding of the pathways of cardiac pain is of prime im-

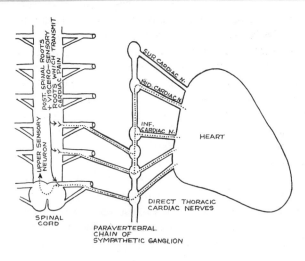

Figure 120. Cardiac pain pathways.

portance in the management of this problem by analgesic block or neurosurgical procedure, since it can be demonstrated that these sensory fibers are conveniently concentrated in the three or four upper thoracic sympathetic ganglia and the four upper thoracic posterior spinal roots. It is at these sites that interruption by block or surgery is best accomplished.

Symptoms and Signs. Anginal pain is usually precordial or substernal, abrupt in onset, and of fairly short duration. It may remain confined to the substernal region or radiate to the shoulders, arms, neck, or back (Fig. 119). Although the most common radiation extends across the left shoulder and arm and down the ulnar aspect of the left forearm and hand, many different patterns of radiating pain may occur. The quality of the pain is variously described in terms of pressure, squeezing, strangling, choking, aching, or tightness. Although the pain is characteristically compelling enough to cause the patient to cease his activities and remain immobile, this is more a reaction to the unpleasant quality of the pain rather than to its intensity. This intensity may vary from fairly mild discomfort to quite severe distress. As a rule the intensity continues to increase until the patient rests or takes nitroglycerin. Most attacks last less than three minutes.

There are no special physical findings that are pathognomonic of this disorder. Although many patients have evidence of cardiovascular disease with arterial hypertension and electrocardiographic and x-ray findings indicating cardiac enlargement, these and other evidences of cardiac damage are indistinguishable from those in other patients of advanced years who do not suffer from this syndrome. Many patients with angina pectoris have a normal life span, but the unpredictable occurrence of serious complications, including sudden death, always renders the prognosis uncertain.

Treatment of Anginal Pain. Most patients with angina pectoris are able to lead a comfortable existence by a restriction of effort within the limits set by the pain and a program of medical therapy. If the patient remains incapacitated in spite of adequate medical measures, special procedures designed for relief of anginal pain should be considered.

When pain relieving measures were first proposed for intractable cardiac pain, it was feared that permanent elimination of anginal pain would deprive the patient of a warning signal and encourage dangerous excesses in activity. Experience has shown that despite the lack of pain, a painless warning signal persists in the form of constriction or dyspnea. The belief that a patient with coronary artery disease would suffer further cardiac damage following extensive denervation of the heart has also been shown to be unfounded.

Stellate Ganglion Block. The inferior cervical sympathetic ganglion frequently blends directly with the first thoracic ganglion or is connected with it by a short segment of the sympathetic trunk. When fused together, the two ganglia are called the stellate ganglion (Fig. 121).

If a patient with intractable anginal pain is subjected to a stellate ganglion block with a local anesthetic, such as procaine or Xylocaine, relief of pain often occurs. In the past, such a favorable result from stellate block was considered an adequate prognostic test and the patient was then subjected to a stellate ganglionectomy. Unfortunately the long-term results of this operative procedure were not so satisfactory as the so-called prognostic block had indicated. Not infrequently the pain in the upper portion of the

161

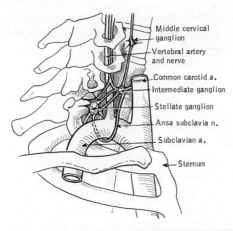

Middle cervical
ganglion

Vertebral artery
and nerve

Common carotid a.

Intermediate ganglion

Stellate ganglion

Ansa subclavia n.

Subclavian a.

Sternum

Figure 121.   The stellate ganglion.

chest was relieved but the residual low precordial pain was a source of considerable discomfort to the patient.

The discrepancy between block and surgery is due to widespread diffusion of the local anesthetic, which involves not only the stellate ganglion but also the upper thoracic ganglia when 10 cc. or more of solution is used. In this instance the term stellate block is misleading; it would be more accurate to refer to this block as a cervicothoracic sympathetic block. The importance of removing the two sympathetic ganglia below the stellate has been documented by White and Sweet in their excellent book on the neurosurgical control of pain. They described several patients who were subjected to stellate ganglionectomy and who continued to complain of low precordial pain. Complete relief of pain occurred only after the second and third thoracic sympathetic ganglia had been removed in a subsequent second surgical procedure.

This block may be helpful in temporarily relieving severe cardiac pain. Since the block is performed with the patient supine, it is easily done without moving the patient from his bed, with no appreciable discomfort, and with an extremely low incidence of complications. The prime disadvantage of this block in the treatment of cardiac pain is the dependence upon the downward diffusion of the anesthetic solution to involve the second and third thoracic ganglia. In many instances the solution does not spread downward as desired. It is possible to infiltrate each ganglion specifically by means of a thoracic paravertebral block. This procedure, however, is not so easily performed and necessitates moving the patient to the x-ray department if x-ray confirmation of proper needle placement is desired. The patient must remain in a prone or lateral position for fairly lengthy periods of time, and the incidence of pneumothorax as a complication of this block is more than negligible. When a local anesthetic is used for temporary relief, the stellate block technique may be given a trial. If one is attempting to obtain a permanent effect from a sympathetic block with the use of alcohol, a more direct needle placement by the posterior paravertebral approach is advisable.

STELLATE BLOCK TECHNIQUE.   With the patient in the supine position, the pillow is removed so that a moderate extension of the head will occur

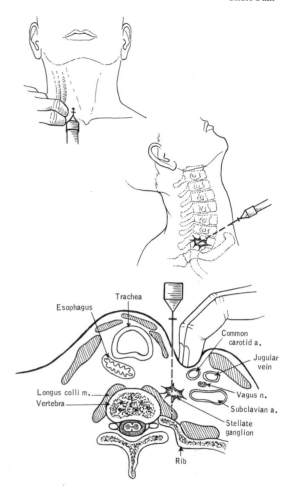

Figure 122. Technique of stellate ganglion block.

(Fig. 122). In short necked individuals, the pillow may be placed under the shoulders to facilitate extension of the head. The neck is palpated, and the carotid artery is pushed laterally while exerting gentle downward pressure to produce a depression between the carotid and the trachea. A skin wheal is made within this depression about 1½ inches above the sternoclavicular joint. A 2½-inch needle, unattached to a syringe, is advanced through the skin wheal with the needle perpendicular to the transverse plane and directed slightly caudad. The needle is advanced posteriorly until bone is contacted. This is the transverse process of the seventh cervical vertebra. At this point the needle has penetrated the longus colli muscle upon which the stellate ganglion lies. To avoid injecting the anesthetic into the belly of this muscle the needle is withdrawn ¼ inch, placing the level just anterior to the muscle and in the same fascial plane as the ganglion. A drop of solution is placed on the hub of the needle to rule out the possibility of pleural penetration. A syringe is then fitted to the needle and aspirated to avoid the remote possibility of penetration of the dura or a blood vessel.

After these precautions have been taken, 10 cc. of anesthetic solution

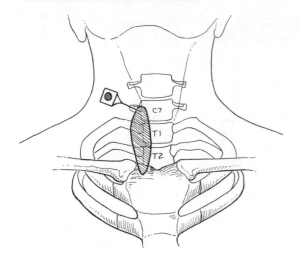

Figure 123.   Elevation of the head permits downward diffusion of the anesthetic agent injected for stellate ganglion block.

is injected. The head of the bed is then elevated to promote diffusion of the anesthetic solution downward to affect the second and third thoracic ganglia (Fig. 123). The site of the pain in the chest and arm determines the side to be blocked. In many cases the predominant pain is left sided and a left stellate block will be effective. When the pain is in the midline or radiates into both upper extremities, bilateral blocks are necessary.

This block may be helpful for control of pain of acute myocardial infarction as well as anginal pain. Because of the ease with which it can be performed in the patient's bed, the block has distinct advantages when moving the patient in and out of bed is contraindicated. If severe chest pain persists in spite of adequate medical management, stellate block may produce very gratifying improvement. Relief of persistent pain is of importance to the general status of a severe infarction, since the feeling of impending doom that accompanies unrelieved cardiac pain may increase emotional stress and anxiety and detrimentally affect the outcome of the disease.

Thoracic Paravertebral Sympathetic Block.   This is the procedure of choice for blocking the thoracic sympathetic ganglia with alcohol in an effort to achieve prolonged relief of cardiac pain (Fig. 124). Although it is quite possible to perform the block in the patient's room while he is lying in his bed, in my opinion it is advisable to carry out this procedure on an x-ray table so that radiographic confirmation of the needle placement can be obtained before injecting a permanent sclerosing solution, such as alcohol. Close cooperation of the anesthesia department is also a source of comfort in the rare case in which respiratory paralysis develops as a complication of this block.

The patient is placed in lateral recumbent position on the x-ray table with the side to be injected uppermost. The legs are drawn up and the head flexed forward in order to obtain a maximal posterior curve of the thoracic spine. To avoid a misleading lateral curvature of the cervical and upper thoracic spine, a thin pillow is adjusted so that the head is supported without lateral deviation. The spinous process of the seventh cervical vertebra is easily identified as the most prominent elevation of the vertebral column. The spinous processes of the thoracic vertebrae are angled downward so that the lamina and body of the first thoracic vertebra lie beneath the spine of the seventh cervical vertebra. This relationship, with the spinous process of the superior vertebra overlying the lamina and body of the vertebra below it, persists over the entire extent of the thoracic spine.

A procaine skin wheal is made 4 cm. lateral to the spinous process of the seventh cervical vertebra and the first, second, and third thoracic vertebrae. A 4-inch, 20-gauge lumbar puncture needle with a depth marker set at 1½ inches is introduced through this wheal perpendicular to the skin and is slowly advanced until the posterior surface of the transverse process is contacted. If the needle is advanced 1½ inches and bone is not contacted, unless the patient is unusually heavy, the needle should be partially withdrawn and redirected to avoid the possibility of inserting the needle between two transverse processes and penetrating the pleura and lung.

When bone is contacted, the depth marker is placed 1¼ inches from the skin. The needle is then withdrawn so that the point is in the subcutaneous tissue and it can be redirected. The needle is now directed medially at an angle of approximately 20 degrees to the median sagittal plane and slightly caudad so that it passes beyond the lower border of the transverse process.

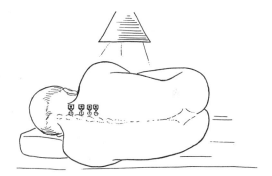

Figure 124. Technique of sympathetic paravertebral block.

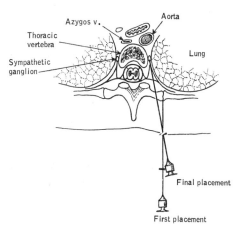

165

In this direction the needle will contact the anterolateral surface of the vertebral body at an added depth of 1¼ inches. If bone is encountered at a depth significantly short of 1¼ inches, the medial angulation of the needle is decreased.

When the first needle is thought to be satisfactorily placed, the stylet is removed from the needle and the three remaining needles are positioned in a similar fashion. The stylet is removed from each needle as soon as it is satisfactorily positioned. This is done to allow time for cerebrospinal fluid or blood to flow out of the needles if they have inadvertently punctured the subarachnoid space or a blood vessel. Elimination of this simple step may lead to an unfortunate mishap, because in some cases spinal fluid or blood cannot be aspirated with a syringe but will slowly flow out of the needle spontaneously. When the needles are properly placed, they are all inserted to the same depth and are parallel to each other in the same plane.

A lateral x-ray of the spine can now be obtained to assure accurate placement of the needles. While the x-ray is being processed, a droplet of procaine is placed on the hub of each needle. This drop should remain undisturbed or may flow slowly through the lumen of the needle. Rapid inspiration of the droplet indicates that the tip of the needle has entered the pleura. Aspiration of each needle is attempted before solution is injected to recheck on the possibility that the needle has perforated a blood vessel or the subarachnoid space. For purposes of diagnosis or therapeutic trial a temporary block can be carried out. Five cubic centimeters of 1 per cent procaine with epinephrine added is injected slowly into each needle. A cough reflex precipitated by the injection indicates penetration of the pleural cavity. The needle should then be withdrawn and if a procaine block is planned, it can be attempted through three well-placed needles in the hope that sufficient diffusion of the procaine will compensate for the absent needle. In performing an alcohol block it is necessary to replace the fourth needle, since alcohol does not diffuse into adjacent tissues so readily as procaine and accurate and complete needle placement is of prime importance. Within five minutes, intercostal anesthesia, an ipsilateral Horner's syndrome, anhidrosis, and an increase in the skin temperature of the ipsilateral upper extremity will occur.

When alcohol is to be used to obtain a long-lasting effect, the initial procaine injection is limited to 2 cc. If a satisfactory sympathetic block is obtained after injection of this limited quantity of solution, it can be assumed that the needles are in close proximity to the sympathetic trunk and an additional 3 cc. of procaine solution can be injected through the needles. This added amount will produce a more widespread anesthesia and prevent pain from the subsequent alcohol injection. Five cubic centimeters of 95 per cent alcohol is injected very slowly through each needle. During the alcohol injection, frequent aspirations are performed to be certain that the tip of the needle has not shifted and penetrated a blood vessel, the subarachnoid space, or the pleura. If the patient complains of discomfort, the injection is halted and the patient examined for any untoward signs. When the discomfort has subsided, the injection is resumed.

At the completion of the procedure, the needles are withdrawn and the patient is maintained in the lateral position for an hour. He may then be transferred from the x-ray table to his bed where he is instructed to lie quietly on his back for several hours. Bed rest is continued until the next morning when he is allowed to walk. Because of the possibility of complications following a thoracic paravertebral injection, it is preferable to keep the patient in the hospital for two or three days after the block.

COMPLICATIONS OF THORACIC PARAVERTEBRAL BLOCK. The complications of this block range from mildly annoying symptoms to death. Pleuritic pain is an occasional annoying complication following an alcohol block and is probably caused by diffusion of the alcohol so that a small amount irritates the pleura. If this pain is to occur, it will be appreciated within several hours after the injection. This is not serious and decreases with symptomatic treatment, including analgesics and adhesive strapping of the chest. Occasionally the pain of pleural irritation may be confused with pneumothorax. This complication results from needle penetration of the pleura and lung, which may produce a bronchopleural fistula that allows alveolar air to be aspirated into the pleural space. The symptoms may vary from mild discomfort in the chest to severe dyspnea and cyanosis. In most cases the use of analgesics, quiet bed rest, and reassurance of the frequently apprehensive patient are all that is necessary. If the symptoms are more severe, it may be necessary to aspirate the air from the pleural space and to administer oxygen. When the diagnosis of pneumothorax is in question, an x-ray of the chest is helpful.

A most serious complication is the injection of local anesthetic or alcohol into the subarachnoid space. Fortunately this is an extremely rare complication but one that the injector must constantly keep in mind. The best way to prevent this occurrence is to use frequent aspirations to make certain that a possible shift of the needle has not allowed the point to enter the subarachnoid space. If procaine or another anesthetic solution is introduced intrathecally, a high spinal anesthesia is produced, the extent of the anesthesia depending upon the quantity of drug injected. If the anesthesia is extensive enough to cause respiratory paralysis, artificial respiration must be instituted promptly and continued until the anesthesia has subsided. In addition to supportive therapy, such as vasopressors to maintain the blood pressure and oxygen, the withdrawal of spinal fluid in large quantities diminishes the amount of anesthetic solution circulating in the cerebrospinal fluid.

I have seen permanent paraplegia and Brown-Séquard paralysis following the inadvertent introduction of alcohol into the subarachnoid space during performance of paravertebral blocks. The effects of alcohol depend as much upon the rapidity of injection as on the amount injected.

A noncritical but troublesome late complication of alcohol block is intercostal neuralgia. The sympathetic ganglia are so close to the intercostal nerves that the latter are invariably affected by the alcohol. Initially they are paralyzed, giving rise to anesthesia, but as the numbness subsides within two to six weeks, discomfort may occur, usually in the form of dysesthesia, tenderness, and burning in the area of the affected dermatomes. This may be treated symptomatically and improves and eventually clears with the passage of time.

Surgical Management of Cardiac Pain. Two surgical procedures are available for sensory denervation of the heart. Posterior rhizotomy, in which the first four thoracic dorsal roots are sectioned bilaterally, assures permanent relief of cardiac pain since interrupted nerve roots will not regenerate.

167

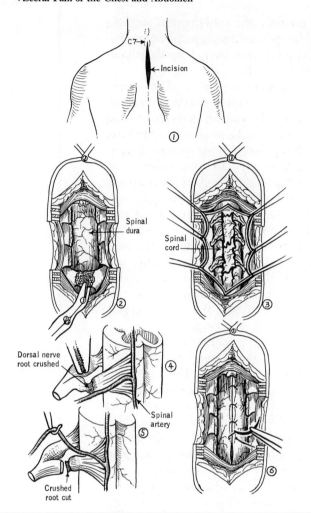

Figure 125. Technique of upper thoracic rhizotomy. (1) Incision. (2) Laminectomy. (3) Retraction of dura. (4) Nerve root crush. (5) Sectioned nerve root. (6) Dural closure.

Another distinct advantage is the opportunity to denervate the cardiac afferent fibers bilaterally, since many patients have pain on both sides of the chest, and occasionally when unilateral chest pain is present after a unilateral sensory denervation has been performed, the pain appears on the contralateral side. The procedure is fairly time consuming, requiring one and a half to two hours. It is usually performed in the prone position, which tends to hamper inspiration, for a relative reduction in the negative intrathoracic pressure impairs the return of blood to the right side of the heart. These are obvious disadvantages to a patient with severe coronary disease. A rare complication of a high bilateral rhizotomy is ischemia of the spinal cord due to interruption of blood vessels that are in close association with the nerve roots and play a role in the vascular supply to the cord. Ordinarily the loss of this blood supply is tolerated without effect, but in the presence of generalized arteriosclerosis the vascular margin of safety to the cord may be reduced.

Resection of the inferior cervical and upper three thoracic sympathetic ganglia is probably the procedure of choice for the patient with unilateral chest and arm pain. Since this procedure can be performed in approximately one hour with the patient in lateral position, it is tolerated fairly well by patients with coronary disease. The possibility of pain's occurring on the contralateral side subsequent to sympathectomy and the occasional regeneration of the sympathetic fibers with recurrence of pain are potential disadvantages. The patient who initially complains of bilateral chest or arm pain would require a bilateral ganglionectomy performed at separate stages, but this procedure probably would involve a greater overall risk than bilateral rhizotomy, which is performed as a single procedure.

TECHNIQUE OF UPPER THORACIC RHIZOTOMY. 1. The skin incision is extended from the seventh cervical (the most prominent spinous process) to the fourth thoracic vertebra. A bilateral subperiosteal muscle dissection is then carried out (Fig. 125).

2. The spines and laminae of the first three thoracic vertebrae are removed. The laminectomy is carried out laterally as far as possible to facilitate subsequent exposure of the nerve roots.

3. The dura is incised in the midline to the upper and lower limits of the bony exposure and retracted by means of stay sutures.

4. The posterior root, which is easily distinguished from the anterior root since it is dorsal to the dentate ligament, is carefully separated from the spinal artery that accompanies the root; the root is then crushed with a hemostat.

5. A fine scissors is used to divide the first four thoracic posterior roots.

6. Closure of dura is performed with interrupted black silk; muscle and fascia are closed with interrupted chromic catgut; and subcutaneous and skin layers are closed with interrupted black silk.

TECHNIQUE OF UPPER THORACIC SYMPATHECTOMY. This procedure can be performed through an incision above the clavicle or by means of the posterior approach, which involves partial resection of the second rib (Fig. 126). The anterior approach may offer considerable difficulty in removing the third thoracic ganglion, especially in patients who are of a stocky, short necked habitus. Since it is important to resect the sympathetic chain down to the third thoracic ganglion, we prefer the posterior approach.

1. The patient is placed in a lateral position with the shoulder slightly forward in order to retract the scapula away from the operative field. The incision is outlined 2 inches lateral to the spinous processes extending from C7 to T4.

2. The trapezius, rhomboid, and serratus posterior superior muscles are divided to expose the second and third ribs. The second rib is easily identified by slipping the finger below the trapezius and rhomboid and over the iliocostalis and longissimus muscles to palpate only a single rib above.

3. The second rib is stripped of periosteum and intercostal muscles to expose a 2-inch segment.

4. This segment of rib is removed, and the protruding transverse process is removed with a rongeur forceps.

5. Through this window into the chest the parietal pleura is gently

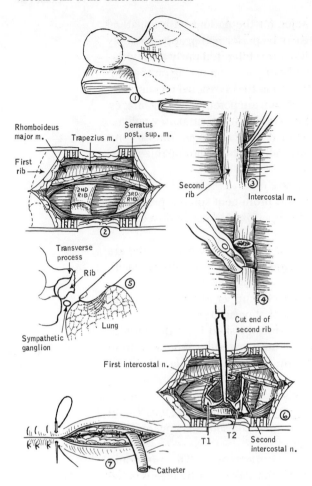

Rhomboideus major m.
Trapezius m.
Serratus post. sup. m.
First rib
Second rib
Intercostal m.
2ND RIB
3RD RIB
Transverse process
Rib
Lung
Sympathetic ganglion
First intercostal n.
Cut end of second rib
T1   T2   Second intercostal n.
Catheter

Figure 126. Technique of upper thoracic sympathectomy.

separated from the sides of the upper four thoracic vertebrae and their attached ribs by finger dissection.

6. The sympathetic chain is now located on the lateral aspect of the exposed vertebra using a lighted retractor to depress the lung if necessary. The chain is first divided below the third ganglion, and then downward traction on the chain is used to expose the stellate ganglion. Silver clips are placed on each ramus before sectioning.

7. Braided wire is used for closure of muscle and fascia and black silk for subcutaneous tissue and skin. A catheter is left within the chest cavity until closure is completed. The anesthetist then increases the pulmonary pressure and the tube is pulled out of the closed incision.

Aortic Aneurysm Pain

Most syphilitic aneurysms of the arch and descending aorta are not associated with severe pain. Occasionally pain from this condition is agonizing, no relief being offered by antiluetic therapy, and the patient not considered suitable for direct surgical attack on the lesion. The size of the aneurysm does not seem to have a direct relationship to pain and the exact cause of pain is uncertain. The pain probably results from a combination of spinal nerve compression related to extensive pressure erosion of adjacent vertebrae and stretching of the wall of the sac and the intrinsic sensory nerve endings in the adventitia of the dilated vessel.

If the patient is a fair operative risk, permanent relief can be offered by posterior rhizotomy, which anesthetizes the total pain area. Many of these individuals, however, are very poor candidates for surgery and cannot tolerate such extensive surgery. In such cases, a procaine block of the upper two thoracic sympathetic ganglia should be performed. This block is frequently effective, because the painful impulses often enter the cord through the sympathetic rami and the sensory axones pass through the upper thoracic ganglia. If pain is relieved by the procaine, the block should be repeated using 95 per cent alcohol.

Pleuritic Pain

Pleurisy or pleuritis is one of the most common causes of chest pain. The parietal pleura is supplied by pain nerve endings whose impulses are transmitted by the intercostal and phrenic nerves. The parenchyma of the lung and its visceral pleura are insensitive to pain.

The exact mechanism producing pleural pain is somewhat in question. A common theory is that pain is created by irritation of the nerve endings due to friction when the two adjacent surfaces are covered with fibrinous exudate. Tension on the inflamed pleural membrane caused by widening of the interspace during inspiration may also produce irritation of the pain nerves within the parietal pleura. Pleuritic pain may occur secondarily to any pulmonary condition that involves the periphery of the lung, such as infection, tumor, or trauma. Involvement of the costal pleura usually causes a rather localized pain in the skin and chest wall overlying the affected area. Mediastinal pleural involvement causes substernal pain, which often radiates to the posterior cervical region and shoulder.

Pain caused by involvement of the diaphragmatic pleura varies according to the site of disease. When it arises in the central portion of the diaphragm, it is referred to the neck and shoulder along the trapezius ridge because of the phrenic innervation. When the source of irritation involves the peripheral portion of the diaphragm, which is supplied by the lower six intercostal nerves, the pain is referred to the lower part of the chest and upper part of the abdominal wall. Since this pain may extend from the xiphoid to below the iliac crest, it is not uncommon for peripheral diaphragmatic pleurisy to be mistakenly diagnosed as cholecystitis and appendicitis.

Treatment. In addition to treatment of the underlying condition, the use of adhesive stripping, local heat, and mild analgesics is usually effective. Occasionally these routine measures are not effective and nerve block therapy is indicated. Intercostal nerve blocks are indicated when involvement of the

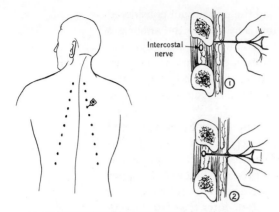

Intercostal
nerve

Figure 127. Technique of intercostal nerve block.

costal pleura or peripheral diaphragmatic pleurisy causes localized chest wall pain.

Technique of Intercostal Nerve Block. The patient is placed in a lateral recumbent position with the side to be injected uppermost for a unilateral block (Fig. 127). For a bilateral block, the patient is placed in a prone position. It is important to place the upper extremity in an adducted position in order to retract the scapula from the area of injection. This is accomplished in the prone position by having the arms hanging over the sides of the table. The angle of the rib, which is the most eminent site of the posterior portion of each rib, is palpated and marked with a cross made by indenting the skin with the fingernail. When obesity makes it difficult to palpate the angle of the rib, the spinous processes of the thoracic vertebrae are used for landmarks. If a mark is made opposite the spinous process, it will approximately correspond to the rib immediately below the selected spinous process. For example, the spinous process of the fourth thoracic vertebra is on the same level as the angle of the fifth rib. A line drawn through the posterior angle of the ribs runs obliquely across the back, the angle of the second rib being 2½ inches lateral to the midline and the tenth, eleventh, and twelfth ribs 4 inches lateral to the midline (Fig. 127 [1]).

A 2-inch, 25-gauge needle is carefully introduced perpendicularly through the skin until the point of the needle contacts the surface of the rib. If a thin needle is used, it is not necessary to make a procaine wheal since the creation of a wheal causes as much discomfort as the introduction of a 25-gauge needle. When the needle is in contact with the bone, the shaft is grasped firmly with the thumb and forefinger ¼ inch from the skin (Fig. 127 [2]). Maintaining this grasp on the needle, the operator withdraws it slightly and moves the overlying skin sufficiently caudad to allow the needle to be reintroduced just beyond the lower border of the rib and advanced as far as the firm grip on the shaft of the needle permits (Fig. 127 [3]). A syringe previously filled with anesthetic solution is adapted to the firmly held needle and aspirated to ascertain whether the point is within the lumen of a blood vessel. If no blood appears, 5 cc. of anesthetic solution is injected. The needle is then withdrawn and the same technique repeated at the next interspace until the area of pain has been adequately blocked.

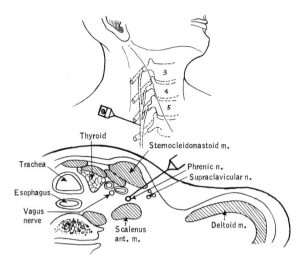

Figure 128. Technique of phrenic nerve block.

If severe intractable pleuritic pain is due to involvement of the central portion of the diaphragm, a unilateral phrenic nerve block may be diagnostically helpful, since this problem is easily confused with other entities. Bilateral phrenic block is not routinely considered because of the associated diaphragmatic paralysis and attendant respiratory dangers.

Technique of Phrenic Nerve Block. The block is performed with the patient in a supine position with the head turned to the opposite side (Fig. 128). A skin wheal is made 1 inch above the clavicle at the posterior border of the sternomastoid muscle. While the index finger retracts the posterior border of the sternomastoid muscle, a 2-inch, 22-gauge needle is introduced in a posteromedial direction beneath the sternocleidomastoid muscle with the point of the needle just above the scalenus anticus muscle, upon which the phrenic nerve courses. Careful aspiration of the syringe is necessary to avoid intravascular injection. Since there are no bony landmarks to serve as a guide, 10 to 15 cc. of solution is required so that the nerve will be blocked by diffusion if not directly.

ABDOMINAL VISCERAL PAIN

Pain Pathways of the Abdominal Viscera

Sympathetic and parasympathetic nerves supply motor fibers to innervate the abdominal viscera. The sympathetic fibers reach the viscera directly or via the greater, lesser, and least splanchnic nerves and are derived from the lower two-thirds of the sympathetic chain. The parasympathetic fibers are supplied by the second, third, and fourth sacral nerves and the vagus nerve.

The sensory nerves that supply the abdomen are not autonomic nerves but are cerebrospinal fibers that merely accompany the splanchnic nerves and the sacral parasympathetics. This may seem confusing, but if it is realized that the myelinated fibers that convey visceral sensation pass in an

173

uninterrupted course through the autonomic ganglia without synapse to reach their cell bodies in the posterior root ganglion, their central processes entering the spinal cord via the posterior root, this classification can be understood readily.

Pancreatic Pain

Pancreatic diseases may cause unbearable, excruciating pain, which characteristically occurs in waves. It is appreciated in the epigastrium and often radiates to the lower thoracic region of the back and occasionally to the costovertebral angles, mainly the left. The pain may be aggravated when the patient lies in the supine position and decreased when he sits or stands. It may be associated with or followed by severe nausea and vomiting, and the unfortunate individual afflicted with this problem may develop malnutrition and generalized wasting. Among the nonmalignant disorders of the pancreas that are frequently associated with pain can be listed acute pancreatitis, chronic pancreatitis, and pancreatic cysts.

Distention and back pressure within the pancreatic duct are presumed to cause the pain. The fibers conveying pain sensation are carried in the right and left splanchnic nerves and the celiac plexus. The right splanchnic trunk transmits pain from the head of the pancreas, and sensation from the tail is conveyed mainly by the left splanchnic trunk. These visceral afferent fibers pursue an uninterrupted course, traversing through the autonomic ganglia to reach the posterior spinal nerve roots and the dorsal root ganglia. They enter into the sixth to the twelfth thoracic nerve roots.

Treatment. The medical and surgical management of the various pancreatic diseases will not be discussed except to note that the accompanying inflammatory changes in the region of the pancreas make a direct surgical attack upon the pancreas a formidable and often dangerous procedure.

When the pain does not respond to the standard methods of therapy, bilateral sympathetic denervation involving excision of a segment of the splanchnic nerves and a ganglionectomy from T9 to T12 is effective in alleviating pain limited to the pancreas. In the presence of inflammatory and fibrotic changes extending well beyond the confines of the pancreas to involve the retroperitoneal branches of the intercostal nerves, sympathectomy is not completely effective. In these instances it is necessary to resort to cordotomy for complete relief of pain.

Analgesic blocks may be helpful as a temporary measure in addition to providing valuable information in predicting the effectiveness of contemplated surgery.

Block of the splanchnic nerves and celiac plexus is probably the most advantageous blocking procedure for intractable pancreatic pain. Although a unilateral block on the side of the pain can be given a trial, effective pain relief is usually obtained only by performing a bilateral block. A complication arising from the bilateral block is the production of widespread splanchnic vasodilatation, creating a signicant drop in blood pressure. This may be of little consequence in young individuals with elastic blood vessels

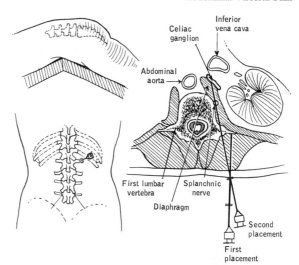

Figure 129. Technique for blocking the splanchnic nerves and celiac plexus.

who are able to partially compensate by vasoconstriction of the unaffected vessels. Elderly patients with generalized arteriosclerosis may not be able to tolerate the precipitous drop in blood pressure. In the presence of arteriosclerosis the likelihood of cerebro- or cardiovascular insufficiency related to the lowered blood pressure is increased. For this reason the block should not be performed unless vasopressors are immediately at hand. One should also be on the alert for postural hypotension subsequent to a bilateral block with syncope and fainting upon assuming the upright position (Fig. 129).

The patient is placed in a prone position with flexion of the lower thoracic and lumbar spine. This can be accomplished with the usual adjustable hospital bed by cranking up the "leg break" and positioning the patient upon this eminence. The spinous process of the first lumbar vertebra is identified by counting up from the first interspace above the iliac crest, which is the L3-L4 interspace.

A skin wheal is made 2 inches lateral to the interspace between the spinous processes of T12 and L1. A 4½-inch, 20-gauge lumbar puncture needle with a depth marker is introduced through the wheal in a perpendicular direction until the point of the needle contacts the transverse process of the first lumbar vertebra at a depth of about 1½ inches. Owing to the caudad slant of the spinous processes the transverse process of L1 is directly below the T12-L1 spinous interspace. The depth marker is then set 2½ inches from the skin, and the needle is withdrawn until its point is in the subcutaneous tissue. The needle is reintroduced in a slightly cephalad and medial direction. This allows the needle to slide over the transverse process of the first lumbar vertebra and impinge upon the lateral surface of the body of the twelfth thoracic vertebra. The needle is slowly advanced, maintaining contact against bone until the depth marker is ¾ inch from the skin at which point contact with the bone ends. At this point the splanchnic nerves are blocked by injecting 10 to 15 cc. of local anesthetic solution. This in most cases is sufficient to give relief of pancreatic pain, and if a lower thoracic

175

ganglionectomy and splanchnicectomy are contemplated for the future, this limited block will be of greater prognostic value than a block of both the splanchnic nerves and the celiac ganglia.

To block the celiac ganglia the needle is then further advanced until the marker is flush with the skin, which places the point of the needle ½ to ¾ inch in front of the anterior surface of the vertebral body. If the placement of the needle is correct, the point is within the retroperitoneal space just anterior to the crus of the diaphragm. It is important to aspirate prior to injecting because the inferior vena cava and aorta, which are just anterior to the needle, increase the likelihood of an accidental intravascular injection. The celiac ganglion can be blocked with the needle in this position using 15 cc. of local anesthetic solution.

A paravertebral block of the sixth to eleventh thoracic ganglia accomplishes a similar result to the spanchnic and celiac block, but the multiple needle placement required is a distinct disadvantage.

Surgery. In cases of pancreatic pain, supradiaphragmatic sympathectomy, in which the ninth to eleventh sympathetic ganglia and a segment of the major splanchnic nerve are excised, is the most advantageous procedure. It is a less extensive operative procedure than the standard thoracolumbar ganglionectomy and splanchnicectomy. These latter procedures are frequently followed by postoperative discomfort due to neuralgia of the twelfth thoracic and first lumbar nerves, which are invariably stretched in the transdiaphragmatic dissection. Another advantage is the feasibility of performing a bilateral procedure at one session if trained assistants are available to carry out the contralateral opening and closure while the surgeon is working on the opposite side.

TECHNIQUE. Under endotracheal anesthesia the patient is placed in a prone position, blanket rolls or pillows assuring freedom of abdominal and respiratory excursions (Fig. 130). (1) A 6-inch incision is made 2 inches lateral to the thoracic spine with the incision centered over the eleventh rib. (2) The iliocostalis dorsi and longissimus dorsi muscles are incised in the direction of their fibers and retracted to expose the eleventh rib. (3) Using a periosteal elevator to denude the intercostal muscles and periosteum from the rib, the operator excises a 2-inch segment of rib, making sure to resect the medial portion of the rib to the transverse process of the eleventh thoracic vertebra. Taking care to avoid opening the parietal pleura, a finger is inserted into the lateral gutter and the pleura is freed from the medial portion of the diaphragm and the lower thoracic vertebrae. (4) A lighted retractor is then used to retract the lung anteriorly. The sympathetic trunk with its ganglia can be identified running over the costovertebral articulations. The greater splanchnic nerve is located more anteriorly on the vertebral bodies and can be followed as it passes through the diaphragm.

(5) The sympathetic chain is resected from the ninth to the eleventh ganglia, dividing the rami communicantes after silver-clipping them; this resection includes the origin of the lesser splanchnic nerve. A 2- or 3-inch segment of the greater splanchnic nerve can then be excised. Interrupted stainless steel wire is used to close the muscle and fascia; interrupted black silk technique is used for the subcutaneous and skin layers. To assure re-

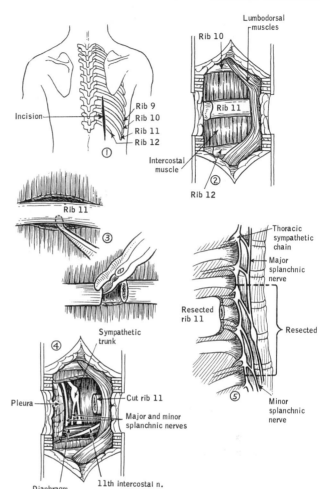

Figure 130. Technique of supra-diaphragmatic sympathectomy.

expansion of the lung, the anesthetist increases pulmonary pressure as the muscles and fascia are sutured. A catheter is left in the retropleural space until closure is completed when it is aspirated with a syringe to remove all air and then withdrawn through the closed incision.

Gallbladder and Biliary Tract Pain

Disease of the gallbladder and adjacent bile passages is a relatively frequent cause of pain in the upper abdominal region. Distention of the gallbladder and the cystic and common bile ducts is the "adequate stimulus" for production of pain. Depending upon the disease involving the gallbladder, the pain may be intermittent or continuous. It is localized in the right upper quadrant and may be associated with pain radiating to the back, usually in the region beneath the right scapula. If the pain is severe, abdominal tenderness, muscle spasm, nausea, vomiting, and anorexia are often present.

177

Pain is mediated by sensory fibers running in plexuses along the biliary ducts. The majority of these fibers are conveyed by the right greater splanchnic nerve and pass directly without synapse to the dorsal ganglia of the seventh and eighth posterior nerve roots. The predominantly right sided pain innervation of the biliary passages is corroborated clinically, although in some cases it is also necessary to block the left splanchnic nerve for complete relief of pain.

Acute cholecystitis, biliary colic, and biliary dyskinesia are generally managed adequately with standard medical and surgical procedures and are not usually considered pain problems. Postcholecystectomy pain, however, is a serious clinical problem, which may be associated with severe and intractable pain that does not respond to standard medical management and may require special pain relieving procedures. The cause of the persistence of pain and other symptoms of biliary dysfunction following cholecystectomy is not definitely known. Operative trauma to the common bile duct and persistence of stones in the common or cystic duct in spite of careful exploration may give rise to postoperative disability. Peptic ulcers, chronic pancreatitis, residual biliary infection, or in fact any intra-abdominal visceral disease may produce reflex biliary dyskinesia. Biliary dyskinesia, which is considered by some to be the paramount factor in the postcholecystectomy syndrome, usually features spasm of the sphincter of Oddi and dystonia of the gallbladder and biliary tract. The formation of scar tissue around the nerve fibers of the biliary system may also play a role in this condition.

Treatment. Intractable gallbladder and biliary tract pain that does not respond to standard medical and surgical therapy should be subjected to a series of analgesic blocks as a therapeutic trial. A right splanchnic block should be performed, and if this does not control the pain promptly, a left splanchnic block should be carried out before effect of the right block has subsided. As a rule either a right or a bilateral splanchnic block proves effective. If repeated blocks are consistently successful in relieving pain, a lower thoracic sympathectomy and splanchnicectomy should be considered if no other approach to the problem appears to be fruitful. It should be fully realized that in many cases this condition involves a severe disorder in gallbladder function in addition to the pain problem. Because of the many factors entering into this situation, sympathetic surgery should be considered only when other means of therapy have been exhausted.

Renal and Ureteral Pain

Distention of the renal pelvis is probably the most common cause of pain arising from the kidney. Distention of the renal capsule may also produce discomfort as does traction upon the renal vessels. The "adequate stimulus" for ureteral pain is smooth muscle spasm or ureteral distention.

The sensory innervation of the kidney and ureter originates from the dorsal root ganglia of the tenth thoracic to the second lumbar nerves. These fibers accompany the lesser and least splanchnic nerves to reach the aorticorenal and celiac ganglia from which sensory fibers form a fine network surrounding the renal vessels and extending to the hilum of the kidney. The substance of the kidney is reached by these sensory fibers via accompanying branches of the renal artery. The sensory innervation to the ureters is derived from the eleventh thoracic to the second lumbar nerves, the fibers terminating in the smooth muscles of the ureter.

Renal-Ureteral Colic. The pain of renal and ureteral colic may be so severe that large doses of opiates fail to provide significant relief of pain. Although infection, neoplasm, and a variety of other conditions may produce renal-ureteral colic, the most common cause of this syndrome and the one most likely to cause excruciating pain is renoureteral lithiasis. In addition to distention of the renal pelvis and ureter as the etiology of pain, reflex smooth muscle spasm of the ureteropelvic junction and ureters may produce a viscious cycle to progressively aggravate and maintain persistence of the pain. The pain may originate in the vicinity of the costovertebral angle, extend across the abdomen, and radiate into the groin and medial aspect of the thigh. Abdominal muscle spasm, nausea, vomiting, and in very severe cases shock are associated. Frequently the patient has a strong desire to urinate, and urination may be extremely painful.

When the standard methods of therapy fail to afford effective relief of pain, nerve block techniques should be considered. Some authorities advocate the use of nerve blocks as a means of reducing the smooth muscle spasm at the ureteropelvic junction and the ureter and in this fashion facilitate the passage of the calculus through the ureter, allowing it to be expelled into the bladder. My personal experience in promoting descent of calculi by means of block therapy has proved disappointing, and although the procedure is based on theoretically sound reasoning I consider it ineffective. Relief of pain, however, can be achieved by block therapy. A paravertebral sympathetic block extending from T10 to L2 or a splanchnic and celiac ganglia block interrupts the sensory innervation of the kidney and ureter.

Renal Pain of Unknown Etiology. The majority of patients who complain of pain that is typically of renal or ureteral origin usually reveal an organic basis for their symptoms if carefully investigated. Occasionally no lesion can be demonstrated by the various diagnostic methods even including, in certain instances, thorough exploration of the kidney at surgery. These problem cases should be carefully evaluated from both a urologic and a psychiatric standpoint. Paravertebral sympathetic block should be used as a diagnostic and prognostic procedure. If a series of blocks is uniformly effective in relieving pain, a placebo block using saline should be performed to determine the role of suggestion in relief of pain. Individuals who respond beneficially to sympathetic block can be subjected to a combined urologic-neurosurgical procedure. Use of the usual thoracolumbar ganglionectomy approach in which the twelfth rib is removed provides a good exposure of the kidney for preliminary exploration. If no renal lesion can be located, the three lower thoracic ganglia and the first lumbar ganglion as well as the splanchnic trunks are resected.

Thoracolumbar Sympathectomy and Splanchnicectomy. The patient is placed in lateral position with the side of the proposed incision uppermost (Fig. 131). It is important to flex the upper thigh and knee to relax the psoas muscle. After the patient is satisfactorily positioned and securely strapped, the middle of the table is angled to increase the space between the

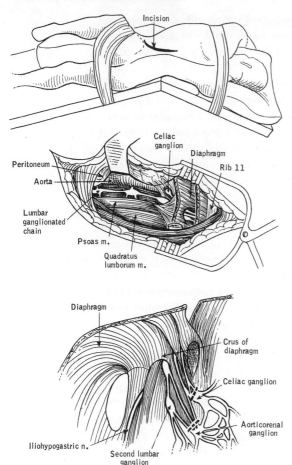

Figure 131. Thoracolumbar sympathectomy and splanchnicectomy.

ribs and the iliac crest. An incision is outlined 2 inches lateral to the spinous processes from the tenth rib down to the upper lumbar region where it then continues in a gentle curve anteriorly to the iliac crest. This incision is carried through the fibers of the trapezius, latissimus dorsi, and sacrospinalis muscles to expose the twelfth rib. The sacrospinalis muscle is retracted toward the spinous processes to expose the central articulation of the twelfth rib, and the entire rib is resected. The transversalis fascia is then incised, and the external and internal oblique muscles are retracted anteriorly exposing the retroperitoneal space.

By careful finger dissection, the peritoneum, kidney, and ureter are separated from the quadratus lumborum and the psoas muscles. The kidney and ureter can then be examined for abnormalities. If no renal lesion can be found, the layer of fat enveloping the renal pedicle is excised carefully to expose the artery and veins with the plexus of nerves surrounding these vessels. These fine nerve fibers are dissected free of the vessels and resected. Although this renal pedicle neurectomy may in itself be adequate to relieve the pain, it is advisable to proceed with a sympathetic ganglionectomy and splanchnicectomy to assure complete interruption of all afferent nerves and to lessen the likelihood of nerve regeneration.

Careful finger dissection is used to free the pleura from the lower thoracic vertebrae, and the diaphragm may be divided to the medial lumbocostal arch to afford a more extensive exposure of the sympathetic ganglia and splanchnic nerves above and below the diaphragm. Lighted retractors are used to retract the pleura to expose the ninth or tenth sympathetic ganglion and the greater splanchnic nerve, which is more deeply located on the anterolateral surface of the vertebral bodies. The greater splanchnic nerve is carefully developed along its course. The sympathetic ganglia are then carefully dissected free of the associated intercostal nerve and artery; silver clips are placed on the communicating rami before they are sectioned.

After the desired lengths of sympathetic chain and greater splanchnic nerve are completely immobilized, they are clipped and resected. The exposure is then carried downward beneath the diaphragm. The greater splanchnic nerve can be identified as it passes through the diaphragm, and 1 or 2 cm. below the diaphragm it merges into the celiac ganglion. The lesser and least splanchnic nerves are found lying between the greater splanchnic and the lumbar sympathetic chains with their fibers parallel to the greater splanchnic. The greater and lesser splanchnic nerves are detached from the celiac ganglion and a segment of the least splanchnic is also resected. The first and second sympathetic chains are then mobilized by freeing up the ganglia and sectioning the communicating rami. It is usually possible to remove the entire sympathetic chain and greater splanchnic nerve in continuity by exerting gentle traction and pulling the subdiaphragmatic portion of the sympathetic trunk of the greater and lesser splanchnic nerves up through the diaphragm.

At the completion of the procedure the divided portion of the diaphragm is carefully approximated using interrupted black silk technique. The muscle layers are closed with interrupted chromic catgut and a catheter is left in the retropleural space. During the closure the anesthetist increases the intratracheal pressure to secure reexpansion of the lung. When all muscles are closed, the catheter is aspirated with a syringe and withdrawn. Skin is closed with interrupted black silk technique.

Pelvic and Perineal Pain

Essential Dysmenorrhea.   Pain associated with menstruation and not related to organic pelvic disease is termed essential or primary dysmenorrhea. This common problem usually has its onset shortly after the menarche but may occur at any age. Uterine ischemia, exaggerated uterine contractions, and other theories have been advanced to explain the mechanism of pain production but the cause remains unknown. An emotional component to this problem has been commonly observed. Daughters of dysmenorrheic mothers, or girls who live with dysmenorrheic relatives, are apt to develop primary dysmenorrhea. These patients are likely to be nervous, unstable women with lowered pain thresholds.

The majority of these problems can be managed adequately with anal-

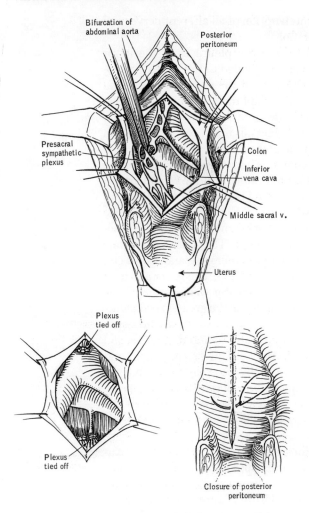

Figure 132.   Presacral neurectomy.

gesics. Postural exercises, endocrine therapy, and cervical dilatations may all be employed in severe cases. In rare instances, when every available form of therapy has failed and the pain is extremely severe and incapacitating, presacral neurectomy should be considered.

Pain from the body of the uterus is conveyed by the superior hypogastric plexus and the preaortic nerves. These afferent fibers enter the spinal cord by means of the eleventh and twelfth thoracic posterior spinal roots. Pain from the uterine cervix is transmitted via sacral parasympathetic fibers to the second, third, and fourth sacral roots.

Technique of Presacral Neurectomy.   With the patient in Trendelenburg position a left paramedian incision is made starting 3 inches above the umbilicus and ending 2 inches above the pubis (Fig. 132). The incision is carried down to the peritoneum, which is incised. With adequate anesthesia supplemented by the Trendelenburg position the coils of the small bowel are easily retracted into the upper abdomen and maintained in position with a moist abdominal pack. The posterior peritoneum is incised in the midline to expose the bifurcation of the abdominal aorta. The incised edges of the posterior peritoneum are retracted with four black silk stay sutures. The superior hypogastric plexus is easily exposed by gently brushing free the retroperitoneal areolar tissue and fat from the lower end of the abdominal aorta and the common iliac vessels. The entire plexus can be retracted gently upward by means of an umbilical tape as the small connecting fibers are cut, for a 2- or 3-inch segment, over the aorta. The main trunks are severed after freeing up a 2- or 3-inch segment over the aorta after which the fibers are followed downward over the sacrum. All bleeding is carefully controlled, and any lymph channels torn should be occluded with silver clips or silk ligatures. The posterior peritoneum is sutured, and the anterior abdominal closure is performed in the usual fashion.

chapter eight —

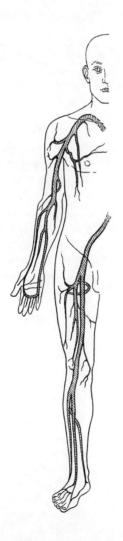

Pain of Peripheral
Vascular Disease

Pain in the extremities secondary to involvement of the peripheral vascular system is a common problem. With the continued increase in our geriatric population, vascular problems, particularly arterial disorders, assume increasing importance. Since localized symptoms of vascular disease are often a manifestation of some generalized condition, an investigation of the pain of peripheral vascular disease must involve in its scope certain factors of major importance relating to the patient as a whole. These factors include generalized arteriosclerosis, hypertension, heart disease, malignant disease, and the presence or absence of diabetes mellitus. The exact nature of the pain must be brought out by careful questioning before effective therapy can be applied. The treatment of rest pain, which is worse at night, is different from that for pain brought on by walking even though both may be caused by the same disease.

RAYNAUD'S DISEASE

In 1862 Maurice Raynaud, a 28-year-old French physician, published a report describing discoloration of the digits after exposure to cold. Included in this publication, moreover, were several case reports that described organic involvement of the major peripheral blood vessels. These undoubtedly have created some confusion so that various experts prefer the term Raynaud's phenomenon and others Raynaud's syndrome instead of Raynaud's disease. As I understand it, the term Raynaud's phenomenon refers to any change in the peripheral circulation that may produce temporary color changes in the digits, including trauma, organic vascular disease, vascular pressure mechanisms, such as the scalenus anticus syndrome, and a variety of systemic diseases, such as scleroderma. Raynaud's disease, on the other hand, is a specific disease entity involving intermittent constriction of the small arteries or arterioles of the extremities in the absence of underlying occlusion of the major arteries, producing color changes in the skin of the digits, such as pallor or cyanosis, with or without local gangrene. These changes are brought on by cold or emotion and are relieved by heat.

The etiology of Raynaud's disease is unknown. The predominance of the disease among women is universally recognized; the ratio of females to males is variously reported as from 5 to 1 to 10 to 1. The highly nervous, underweight, asthenic female appears to be affected most frequently. The onset usually occurs after puberty and before the age of 40 although it may occur at any age. A familial predisposition has been noted, although, in the strict sense of the word, the disease cannot be considered hereditary.

Symptoms and Signs

Color changes in the skin of the digits caused by exposure to cold or emotional stress are the primary symptoms. The fingers initially become blanched, and this is usually followed by a phase of cyanosis in which they become deeply blue. The digits are cold and somewhat numb, and if the phase of cyanosis is prolonged, there is impairment of all discrete finger movements associated with pain. This pain may not be particularly severe but may be described as an aching, burning, "pins and needles" sensation or a feeling of tightness. The attack may subside spontaneously or can be terminated if the patient goes into a warm room or immerses the hands in warm water. With subsidence of the attack the cyanotic digits gradually become hyperemic until they are brilliantly red throughout. Initially the episodes may be unilateral but they eventually become bilateral. The onset of these attacks is usually gradual, occurring in the winter and progressively increasing in severity.

When the condition has been present for several years, trophic changes develop. The skin of the digits becomes smooth, shiny, and tightly stretched. The nails develop ridges. Discrete areas of local cutaneous gangrene may appear on the finger tips. In approximately half of all cases of Raynaud's disease only the hands are affected; both hands and feet are affected in the remainder of the patients. The disease progressively worsens in approximately one-third of all cases while in the remainder the disease may persist indefinitely in a mild form or even improve spontaneously. In common with all peripheral vasospastic conditions, the disease tends to improve or disappear during pregnancy and worsens during the menstrual period or at the menopause.

Pathology

Mildly ill patients and those in the early stages of the disease reveal no abnormalities. In long-standing, progressive cases the small arteries in the digits reveal intimal thickening and hypertrophy of the muscular coat, which eventually may lead to thrombosis and areas of focal gangrene. Even severe cases show no change in the large vessels of the extremities.

Treatment

A large number of these patients respond to avoidance of exposure of the body, as well as the extremities, to cold. Abstinence from smoking does not appear to provide discernible benefit in most cases, although it should be given at least a reasonable trial. The various vasodilating drugs should also be given a trial but usually are disappointing. The emotional component of this condition should be recognized and should receive considerable attention. Most patients become extremely apprehensive regarding the likelihood of the development of gangrene, and reassurance is important that this eventuality will not occur if the patient can be followed at close intervals. Sedatives, tranquilizers, and supportive psychotherapy are of utmost importance.

When the attacks are frequent and severe and are accompanied by significant pain, regional sympathectomy is indicated. The results of lumbar sympathectomy, excising L2 and L3 are good in approximately 90 per cent of cases. Thoracic sympathectomy (T1 to T3) is effective in about 70 to 75 per cent of cases involving the hands.

Technique of Lumbar Sympathectomy.   Under spinal anesthesia, the patient is placed in a semisupine position with a cushion under the side of surgery (Fig. 133). The knee on the side of surgery is flexed to relax the psoas muscle. A skin incision corresponding to the course of the external oblique fibers is extended from the costal margin for a distance of 6 inches to a point below the anterior superior iliac spine. The muscles of the anterior abdominal wall are split in the direction of their fibers until the peritoneum is encountered. At this point, using careful finger dissection to avoid opening the peritoneum, the peritoneum is carefully dissected free from the inner surface of the quadratus lumborum until the lateral margin of the psoas muscle is encountered. It is important not to dissect between the quadratus lumborum and the psoas muscle. Usually this line of cleavage is established readily and the fingers contact the anterolateral portion of the second lumbar vertebra; often the sympathetic chain can be palpated.

Deep retractors are used to retract the peritoneum medially, and the lumbar sympathetic chain is exposed in the junction between the psoas muscle and the anterior portion of the vertebra. On the right side the vena cava may lie over the sympathetic chain, and in retracting this structure due care is taken to prevent a rent in the relatively thin wall. The vena cava occasionally can create a problem if previous surgery has created adhesions in the area. It is important to clip or cauterize the numerous bridging vertebral veins, which occasionally pass over the right sympathetic trunk. These lumbar vessels do not usually present so great a problem on the left side, and the aorta is not in a position to compromise the exposure.

The sympathetic chain is elevated by a nerve hook, which facilitates exposure of the communicating rami; these are divided. No difficulty is encountered in removing the second and third lumbar ganglia. In order to expose the first lumbar sympathetic ganglion it is necessary to incise the crus of the

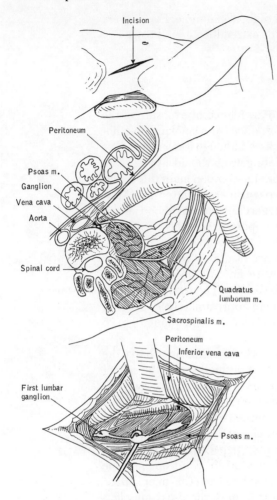

Incision

Peritoneum

Psoas m.
Ganglion
Vena cava
Aorta

Spinal cord

Quadratus
lumborum m.

Sacrospinalis m.

Peritoneum
Inferior vena cava

First lumbar
ganglion

Psoas m.

Figure 133. Technique of lumbar sympathectomy. In positioning the patient, it is advantageous to flex the knee on the side of surgery in order to relax the psoas muscle.

diaphragm. However, for vasospastic problems involving the foot and leg, it is not necessary to excise above the second lumbar ganglion. The usual closure of the anterior abdominal muscle splitting incision is performed in layers.

Technique of Upper Thoracic Sympathectomy. The posterior approach described in the section on cardiac pain (p. 169) can be used. For sympathetic denervation of the upper extremity, I generally prefer the anterior or supraclavicular exposure. This approach is satisfactory for excision of the first, second, and third thoracic ganglia, and it is usually associated with considerably less postoperative discomfort than the more extensive posterior approach, which involves removal of the second rib and division of several large muscles (Fig. 134).

Under endotracheal anesthesia, the patient is placed in a supine position with the neck slightly extended and the head rotated toward the opposite shoulder. (1) An incision is made a thumbsbreadth above and parallel to the clavicle, starting over the clavicular insertion of the sternocleidomastoid muscle and carrying it laterally about 8 cm. (2) The platysma muscle is divided, exposing the tendon of the sternocleidomastoid muscle with its attachment to the clavicle. (3) The clavicular portion of the sternocleido-mastoid muscle is divided, exposing the omohyoid muscle, which is also divided.

At this point, the scalenus anticus muscle, which is stretched taut by the position of the head and neck, can be palpated easily as a firm bundle of muscle fibers. (4) The fat and fascia overlying the scalenus anticus muscle are carefully dissected to identify the phrenic nerve, which runs obliquely across the muscle from the lateral to the medial borders. When this pro-cedure is carried out on the left side, the fatty tissue above and medial to the scalenus anticus muscle is retracted medially with the phrenic nerve to avoid injury to the thoracic duct. (5) A knife or scissors is used to divide the musculotendinous insertion of the muscle in small groups of fibers, which retract upward as they are sectioned, exposing the uncut fibers. When the

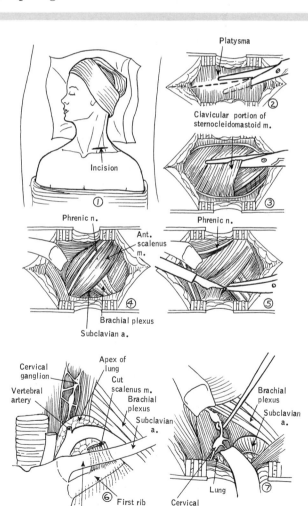

Figure 134. Supraclavicular exposure for upper thoracic sympathectomy. The sixth drawing indicates the anatomic relation-ships of the area and is not intended to represent the structures visualized at sur-gery.

scalenus anticus muscle is divided completely, the arch of the subclavian artery and the lateral portion of the brachial plexus can be seen (6, 7).

The dissection is carried out medial to and above the subclavian artery. At this point it is usually necessary to ligate the costocervical trunk or a branch of the thyrocervical trunk to facilitate the exposure. Upon developing the dissection medially, the pleura and the vertebral artery are exposed. A fibrous aponeurosis, known as Sibson's fascia, which arises from the scalenus minimus muscle and connects with the inner surface of the first rib, helping to support the cupola or the apex of the pleura, must be divided by careful blunt dissection. The stellate ganglion is identified behind the vertebral artery, and by continuing the dissection downward it is possible to expose the second and third ganglia and occasionally the fourth ganglion in long-necked individuals. The sympathetic chain is excised in the usual fashion by first dividing the communicating rami and then the chain itself in one continuous length. At the completion of the procedure the divided portion of the sternomastoid muscle is reapproximated using chromic catgut. The remainder of the closure can be performed in layers using interrupted black silk technique. No attempt is made to resuture the scalenus anticus muscle.

TRENCH FOOT

Injury to the foot and lower extremity resulting from prolonged exposure to low temperatures combined with persistent dampness was extensively described during World War I as trench foot. A similar if not identical condition involving amphibious and maritime hazards during World War II was labeled immersion foot. In addition to prolonged exposure to cold, the following conditions are important in the development of this condition: immobility and dependency of the lower extremities, prolonged dampness or actual immersion in cold or cool water, exhaustion, and dehydration. All these conditions tend to reduce the blood flow to the extremities. In some instances deficient intake of proteins and vitamins is an important contributing factor.

Trench foot or immersion foot can be produced in laboratory animals by prolonged immersion of the extremities in cold water. Such immersion causes persistent local tissue anoxia, which, when combined with cold, produces capillary wall damage. This in turn allows the passage of plasma into the tissue spaces, causing edema, which further embarrasses the peripheral circulation. These changes progress to desquamation of the skin, ischemic neuritis with wallerian degeneration, fibrosis of muscle fibers, and, in severe cases, gangrene.

Symptoms and Signs

The initial vasospastic ischemic phase persists as long as the extremity is subjected to a cold, damp environment and the body is exposed to cold. In addition to direct vasoconstriction of the superficial arteries and arterioles, there are undoubtedly reflex vascular changes due to lowering of the body temperature with cooling of the circulating blood. The condition develops quite insidiously with numbness and a mild "pins and needles" sensation signaling the onset. As long as the tissues are supported by boots, the slight swelling of the extremities may not be noted. When the boots are removed, a rapidly developing edema occurs accompanied by paresthesia and severe pain. Arterial pulsations are reduced and often absent. The skin, which is red initially, becomes a cadaveric, pale, mottled, yellow or cyanotic color. Stocking anesthesia or hypesthesia to touch and pin prick is present.

After the patient has been removed from the cold and placed in a warmer environment, the hyperemic stage occurs. Within several hours the feet become red, hot, and dry with bounding peripheral pulses. Tissue swelling increases and blisters appear, filling with serous or hemorrhagic fluid. Ulceration and gangrene may occur in areas of skin supplied by thrombosed vessels. The stocking anesthesia diminishes and is replaced by intense paresthesias of a burning nature, which may be associated with severe lancinating pains. In mild cases the stage of hyperemia subsides in several days and the circulation may become normal with restoration of normal skin tone and temperature. In severe cases the phase of hyperemia persists for several weeks and is followed by paresthesia, pain, coldness, and cyanosis of the lower extremities with or without gangrene. The persistent indurated swelling associated with this late vasospastic ischemic phase may progress to fibrosis, limited joint motion, and deformity. Exposure to cold may provoke a typical Raynaud's phenomenon, and this increased sensitivity to cold may persist for years after the initial episode.

Treatment

This problem is encountered most frequently in military combat or marine disaster, the exigencies of the situation often making preventive measures difficult. However, an understanding of the value of foot hygiene in warfare has led to a sharp decrease in the number of individuals afflicted with this disease. Thick warm socks should be worn, and when these become wet they should be replaced by a dry pair if possible. Any constriction to the circulation, such as circular garters and tight leggings, should be avoided. In World War II and the initial phase of the Korean campain, the incidence of trench foot was high when front line soldiers wore the tight fitting, paratroop style leather boot. As a neurosurgeon within the combat zone during the Korean engagement, I had the opportunity to see the incidence of trench foot diminish sharply with the use of the so-called "vacuum bottle" type of boot. This somewhat ungainly but comfortably roomy foot gear utilized waterproof inner and outer layers separated by a spongy insulating layer.

When the patient is seen during the stage of hyperemia, the aim of treatment is to keep the metabolism of the extremity at a relatively low level and to protect the already insulted and hypervulnerable tissues from further damage by trauma or infection. The patient is placed at strict bed rest, and the feet are moderately elevated above the level of the heart to aid in control and removal of edema. Trauma of any degree is avoided, including massage, and the formation of pressure ulcers, which are particularly common on the heels, is avoided by the use of sponge rubber pads appropriately placed. A cradle is used to prevent the bed covers from traumatizing involved tissues. If tissue damage is present, antibiotics are administered until the danger of bacterial infection has subsided. The body may be covered with blankets, but it is advisable to keep the affected extremities exposed to room temperature (70° F. is optimal).

In severe cases with development of a late vasospastic ischemic phase, active and passive exercises, gentle massage, and mild heat are helpful. If gangrene occurs, early debridement or amputation is to be avoided. Once spontaneous demarcation has occurred, it is often gratifying to find that the deeper structures are viable. I have been happily surprised on several occasions to see what was originally thought to be a most extensive area of gangrene eventually confine itself to the skin alone and separate spontaneously, revealing healthy deep tissues that were suitable for skin grafting.

Patients who manifest persistently severe sensitivity reactions to cold may find it necessary to move to a warmer climate. Frequently this cold sensitivity diminishes in one or two years. When the arterial circulation remains inadequate, a lumbar sympathectomy is indicated.

FROSTBITE

Frostbite is actual freezing of the tissues resulting from exposure to temperature usually below −13° C. (10° F.). Occasionally higher temperatures may produce frostbite if augmented by dampness, strong winds, general body chilling, or any peripheral vascular disturbance of the ischemic type. It is not known whether the prime factor is the formation of ice crystals in the tissues or whether the changes that occur in blood vessels are responsible for the tissue damage.

Signs and Symptoms

The first sign of frostbite may be the development of a white, numb area of hard skin. A painful "pins and needles" sensation is often associated with this phenomenon, or the cold may produce rather complete numbness and anesthesia so that the freezing may be painless. The local tissue injury resulting from frostbite ranges from transient anesthesia and yellowish white discoloration of the skin to persistent ischemia, secondary thrombosis, deep tissue destruction, and gangrene.

Treatment

Frostbite is preventable and rarely occurs in individuals trained to protect themselves properly against the cold. If the early stages of frostbite can be recognized, the problem can be managed easily by covering the area with clothing or a warm body surface until circulation is reestablished. The affected area should not be massaged or rubbed with snow.

In more advanced degrees of frostbite the frozen tissues should be re-warmed as rapidly as can be accomplished by immersing them in water heated to 42° C. (108° F.). When thawing has occurred, immersion is discontinued and complete bed rest is instituted with the frozen region exposed to the room air at 20° C. (70° F.). Antibiotic therapy is of value for prophylaxis against secondary infections if local damage is extensive. Opiates may be necessary for alleviation of pain. Early heparinization to combat thrombosis and gangrene is of equivocal benefit; cortisone and ACTH are of no value. When gangrene is present, the areas affected may be more superficial than was originally apparent so that amputation should not be performed precipitously.

Sympathetic blocks or sympathectomy is not of value, in my experience, in the initial phases of frostbite. If a syndrome of hypersensitivity to cold, vasospasm, and paresthesia results as a late sequel to frostbite, sympathectomy may be of some benefit. Intractable pain as a late symptom is not so common with frostbite as it is in immersion foot.

THROMBOANGIITIS OBLITERANS

Thromboangiitis obliterans, or Buerger's disease, is an inflammatory obliterative disease chiefly affecting the peripheral arteries and veins and occurring almost exclusively in young and middle aged males. The specific etiology is unknown, and it is possible that several different factors may be individually responsible for provoking the pathologic response of this condition in individuals who may be sensitive to a certain toxin or agent. The use of tobacco, particularly cigarettes, causes an obvious pernicious effect upon the progress of the disease. Hemoconcentration and an increased tendency to coagulation of the blood have been found in many cases of thromboangiitis obliterans. Various bacteria have been cultured from cutaneous lesions, and infection or the activity of a toxic agent resulting from infection has also been considered a factor in the etiology of this condition.

All races are subject to thromboangiitis obliterans, but the disease appears to be slightly more common among Jews. Although verified cases have been reported in females, the disease occurs predominantly in males in a ratio of 75 to 1. The clinical manifestations of the disease usually appear between the ages of 20 and 45 years.

Pathology

The pathologic picture of thromboangiitis obliterans is characteristic and distinct from that of other vascular lesions. The lesions are segmental with involved sections of arteries or veins separated by areas that are still normal. Cellular proliferation of the intima in the acute stage is followed by the

193

formation of a red thrombus. The wall of the involved vessel is infiltrated by polymorphonuclear leukocytes and lymphocytes with eventual cellular extension into the thrombus, which becomes organized by means of a heavy growth of fibroblasts in a comparatively short time. Eventually the occluded artery, vein, and contiguous nerves are bound inseparably into a bundle of hard fibrous cords. The unaffected segments of artery and vein are eventually involved at varying intervals so that a single length of artery may exhibit various stages of the disease process ranging from cellular proliferation of the intima to dense scar formation. Occlusion of the arteries is followed by enlargement and development of collateral and anastomotic vessels. Minor recanalization of partly organized thrombi may aid the enlarged collateral vessels in restoring peripheral circulation.

For reasons not completely clear to me, the incidence of Buerger's disease appears to be declining. This in turn has created a certain skepticism regarding the validity of the diagnosis of thromboangiitis obliterans. I believe the early concepts of Buerger's disease may have been looser and not so strictly defined as they are today. Many individuals with arterial insufficiency and intermittent claudication of the lower extremities with onset of symptoms before the age of 45 would have been classified automatically as Buerger's disease some years ago and are now labeled as early cases of atherosclerosis.

Symptoms and Signs

The disease is manifested by an irreguar, relapsing course with periods of arterial occlusion and local tissue injury alternating with quiescent periods during which the collateral circulation assumes some of the function of the occluded vessels. The relationship between vascular occlusion and compensation determines whether the course of the disease will be rapid or slow. As a rule vascular occlusion slowly overextends the compensatory collateral circulation, and several years after the initial mild symptoms are manifested, definite peripheral ischemia becomes established.

The symptoms are due to impairment of the arterial blood supply to tissues and to injury or infection of ischemic tissues. Initially the patient may complain of a sensation of coldness involving the lower extremities. Intermittent claudication with an aching pain commonly appreciated in the arch of the foot and the calf of the leg after exercise may occur in any stage of the disease. The pain of intermittent claudication subsides promptly with rest. Skin color changes, such as cyanosis or redness, may be observed during the course of the illness. Small ulcers are likely to occur on the digits as the result of minor trauma, such as the pressure of the shoes when walking, excessive heat, or irritating local medication. A not infrequent precipitating cause of this initial ulcer is the ill advised removal of corns or ingrown toenails. These small digital ulcerations, which would heal rapidly in a normal individual, extend, and gangrene usually develops.

Severe persistent pain is appreciated in the ulcerative and gangrenous region and the digits. This "rest pain" is usually worse at night, is constant, and is often described as an aching, burning sensation. The gangrene is usually asymmetric and begins as a dark discoloration of the skin, which eventually becomes mummified and dark brown or black. Late in the course of the disease the severe and widespread pain of ischemic neuropathy occurs. This is usually associated with a variety of paresthesias, including "pins and needles," tingling, and crawling sensations, and is paroxysmal. The pain may follow the distribution of an involved peripheral nerve and is lancinating, often described as electric shock-like. This pain offers a problem in treatment, for it does not usually respond to the standard analgesics.

Examination reveals reduced or absent pulsations in the posterior tibial and dorsalis pedis arteries, the popliteal and femoral pulsations usually being normal. Palpation reveals coldness of the involved limb. Elevation of the extremity produces pallor, and there is usually a significant delay before the color returns to the skin with dependency. This delay, which may vary from 15 to 60 seconds or longer, is an approximate indication of the degree of ischemia. The degree of trophic changes and muscle wasting also depends on the duration and severity of peripheral ischemia. Initially the disease severely affects one extremity, while the relatively unaffected side may manifest some degree of vasospasm and possibly mild organic arterial occlusion. The lower extremities are usually involved. However, the disease has been reported in the small arteries of the hands and in the coronary, cerebral, mesenteric, and renal arteries. X-rays may reveal necrosis of bone in an area of ulceration or gangrene; they also often demonstrate osteoporosis in advanced cases.

Treatment

The severity and progressiveness of thromboangiitis obliterans varies, but eventually a stage may be reached when the formation of new occlusive arterial lesions stops. The goal of treatment is to minimize tissue destruction and loss until this stage is reached and the prognosis improves. A diagnosis made early in the course of the disease offers greater likelihood of instituting preventive measures before irreversible tissue damage develops.

Exposure to cold should be avoided as much as possible; warm clothing, fleece lined gloves, and shoes should be worn routinely. Work that requires prolonged standing and walking or exposure to winter weather is detrimental, and if at all possible an indoor sedentary occupation should be sought. The skin should be kept clean and dry, and minor surgery or other trauma should be avoided.

Every patient with thromboangiitis obliterans must give up completely the use of tobacco. Medications such as tranquilizers or sedatives are not especially helpful in solving the smoking problem. A clear understanding of the potential disaster that may result from even an occasional cigarette is the strongest means of discouraging smoking. Neither the physician nor the patient may compromise on this point.

Thrombophlebitis associated with thromboangiitis obliterans presents a problem in management. Anticoagulant therapy with Dicumarol or other common anticoagulants may be of use to avoid propagation and to prevent the rare occurrence of pulmonary embolism. If edema is present, warm

195

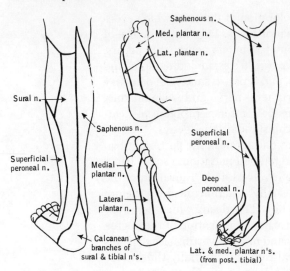

Figure 135. Peripheral nerve sensory fields of foot and leg.

packs and moderate elevation can also be utilized. However, local external heat should be used only with greatest caution because of the danger of blistering and burning.

The pain of infection is severe, occurs at rest, and requires absolute bed rest. The affected extremities should not be elevated but should be maintained either horizontal or slightly (20 degrees) below horizontal since the dependent position aids peripheral blood flow. The extremities should be inspected daily for lesions resulting from pressure or friction of sheets or bed clothes. Infected lesions are treated by moist dressings and topical applications of antibiotic agents. Systemic antibiotic therapy should also be utilized. In treating infections, strong antiseptics are best avoided because of the danger of injuring tissues already partially devitalized. The rest pain may require analgesics ranging from aspirin to morphine. When the pain is intractable, the alcoholic injection or the crushing of peripheral nerves produces anesthesia of two to six months' duration.

Technique of Peripheral Nerve Block. The area of pain determines the nerve to be blocked. In many instances the pain is rather widespread and involves an area supplied by several nerves. The site of maximal pain should be attacked initially in the hope that the surrounding pain is merely a radiating dysesthesia. This is more likely to be true when the site of maximal pain coincides with a destructive lesion, such as an ulcer or gangrene (Fig. 135).

Saphenous Nerve Block. The saphenous nerve, which arises from the posterior division of the femoral nerve, is the largest cutaneous branch from the femoral nerve and may be regarded as the terminal branch of that nerve. It originates from the femoral nerve in the femoral triangle and becomes superficial by passing between the sartorius and gracilis muscles on the medial aspect of the knee. It supplies the skin over the medial, anteromedial, and posteromedial aspects of the leg, extending from the knee to the ball of the great toe.

The skin wheal is raised on the medial aspect of the knee just below the inferior border of the patella (Fig. 136). A 25-gauge, 1½-inch needle is inserted perpendicularly through the skin and advanced until paresthesia is elicited along the saphenous nerve. If bone is contacted before paresthesia is elicited, the needle is partially withdrawn and redirected until the nerve is contacted. One cubic centimeter of 95 per cent alcohol is slowly injected after aspirating the syringe to be certain that the saphenous vein, which is adjacent to the nerve, has not been entered.

Superficial Peroneal Nerve Block. The superficial peroneal nerve begins at the bifurcation of the common peroneal nerve between the neck of the fibula and the proximal part of the peroneus longus muscle. It continues downward in the intermuscular septum between the peronei and the extensor digitorum longus muscle. It pierces the deep fascia at the junction of the middle and lower thirds of the leg at which point it divides into two terminal branches. The nerve supplies the skin of the dorsum of the foot and the dorsal surface of the toes with the exception of the adjacent sides of the first

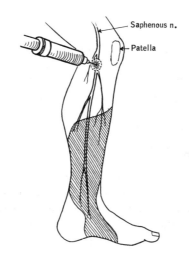

Figure 136. Saphenous nerve block.

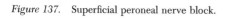

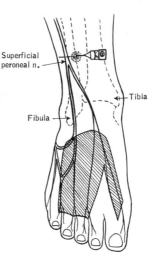

Figure 137. Superficial peroneal nerve block.

197

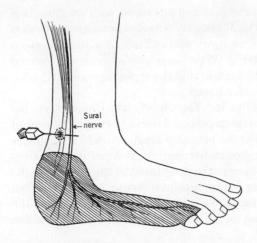

Sural
← nerve

Figure 138.   Sural nerve block.

and second toes (deep peroneal nerve) and the lateral side of the fifth toe (lateral dorsal cutaneous branch of the sural nerve).

A wheal is made 5 inches above the ankle joint at a point midway between the anterior border of the tibia and the lateral border of the fibula (Fig. 137). A 2-inch, 25-gauge needle is slowly introduced through the wheal at such an angle that the point of the needle is directed toward the lateral aspect of the fibula. If paresthesia is appreciated, 1 cc. of alcohol is slowly injected through the needle. In the absence of paresthesia, 10 cc. of 2 per cent procaine solution is slowly injected as the needle is withdrawn. It may be necessary to crush the nerve under direct vision.

Sural Nerve Block.   The sural nerve is a terminal sensory nerve of the common peroneal nerve. The lateral sural cutaneous nerve arises from the common peroneal nerve in the popliteal fossa. It becomes superficial by piercing the deep fascia over the lateral head of the gastrocnemius and extends to the middle third of the leg where it joins the anastomotic branch of the tibial nerve to form the sural nerve. It supplies sensation to the lateral aspect (distal third) of the leg and to the ankle and heel.

A wheal is raised 1 inch above the heel and on the lateral edge of the Achilles tendon. A 1-inch, 25-gauge needle is introduced through the wheal with a slight lateral angulation. At a depth of ½ to ¾ of an inch, paresthesia of the sural nerve may be appreciated (Fig. 138).

Posterior Tibial Nerve Block.   The tibial nerve is the larger of the two terminal branches of the sciatic nerve. One of its terminal branches, the posterior tibial nerve, begins at the distal border of the popliteus muscle and courses downward in the leg in the sheath that separates the deep and superficial muscles of the leg. In the ankle, it lies close to the posterior aspect of the tibia and is accessible for blocking at the medial border of the Achilles tendon just above the malleoli. It lies in close approximation to the artery so that care must be exercised to avoid intravascular injections when it is blocked.

A wheal is made 1 inch above the level of the malleoli on the medial border of the Achilles tendon (Fig. 139). A 2-inch, 25-gauge needle is introduced through the wheal and slowly advanced anteriorly until paresthesia is elicited. If the posterior aspect of the tibia is encountered without paresthesia, the needle is partially withdrawn and redirected slightly more lateral until it impinges upon the nerve. The block will cause analgesia of the side of the foot and paralysis of the plantor muscles.

Saphenous Nerve Crush at the Knee. Under local anesthesia, a 2-inch longitudinal incision is made through the skin and subcutaneous tissue on the medial aspect of the knee one-third above and two-thirds below the inferior portion of the patella (Fig. 140). No difficulty should be encountered in locating the long saphenous vein, which is quite prominent in this region and may even be identified before making the incision. The saphenus nerve can be identified by its close proximity to the vein. The greatest problem encountered in identification of this and other superficial sensory nerves is the tendency to make the initial incision too deep and carry the dissection beneath the proper plane. At this site the nerve lies above the deep fascia. The nerve is crushed with a hemostat and the incision closed, using interrupted black silk technique in two layers.

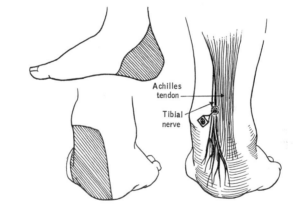

Figure 139. Posterior tibial nerve block.

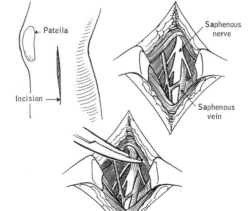

Figure 140. Saphenous nerve crush at the knee.

199

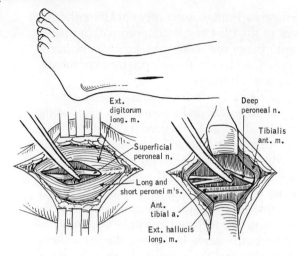

Figure 141. Superficial and deep peroneal nerve crush.

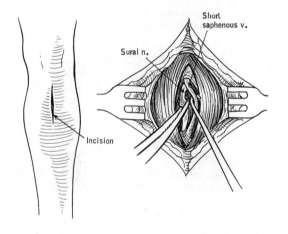

Figure 142. Sural nerve crush.

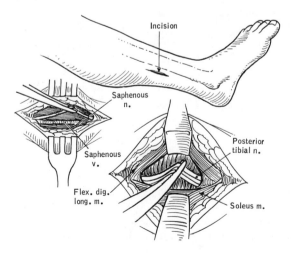

Figure 143. Saphenous and posterior tibial nerve crush.

Superficial and Deep Peroneal Nerve Crush.   Through the same incision it is possible to expose the superficial and deep peroneal nerves (Fig. 141). A 3-inch incision is made under local anesthesia in the lateral aspect of the leg 5 or 6 inches above the external malleolus. The fascia overlying the intermuscular septum between the long and short peronei on the lateral side and the extensor digitorum longus on the medial side is incised. The superficial peroneal nerve is evident just beneath the fascia, lying in the line of cleavage of these muscle fibers. A hemostat is used to crush the nerve.

To expose the deep peroneal nerve, a retractor is used to pull the skin medially, and a line of cleavage is developed between the extensor hallucis longus and the tibialis anterior muscles. This exposes the deep peroneal nerve closely associated with the anterior tibial artery and vein. Care is taken not to injure the artery when crushing the nerve with a hemostat.

Sural Nerve Crush.   The course of the sural nerve is subject to considerable variation. The nerve is best identified by means of a 2-inch incision made under local anesthesia approximately 8 or 9 inches above the heel in the midportion of the calf (Fig. 142). The short saphenous vein can be identified easily within the raphe of the gastrocnemius muscle, and just lateral to the vein the sural nerve can be identified. The nerve is crushed with a hemostat and the wound is closed, using interrupted black silk technique.

Saphenous and Posterior Tibial Nerve Crush.   The same incision enables the saphenous and posterior tibial nerves to be exposed (Fig. 143). A 3-inch incision is made under local anesthesia 5 inches above the internal malleolus. The long saphenous vein is identified lying over the fascia, and adjacent to the vein is the saphenous nerve. The nerve is crushed with a hemostat. The overlying fascia is incised and a plane of cleavage developed between the flexor digitorum longus and the soleus muscles. This exposes the posterior tibial nerve, artery, and vein. The nerve is crushed with a hemostat.

Sympathectomy.   Bilateral lumbar sympathectomy should be considered for the patient with chronic ischemia. Patients with organic arterial occlusion who do not respond to medical treatment may be benefited by the permanent vasodilatation resulting from this surgery. Mild cases with only slight arterial impairment may not require sympathectomy, and in advanced cases with extensive gangrene nothing can be gained. Lumbar sympathetic blocks used to determine the potential value of anticipated surgery are not particularly helpful, since the duration of the block is too short to reproduce the effects of surgery.

ARTERIOSCLEROSIS OBLITERANS

The commonest cause of arterial occlusion is arteriosclerosis obliterans. Mönckeberg's sclerosis, senile gangrene, and diabetic gangrene all fall into this general classification. The disease may affect relatively short portions of the aorta, iliac, femoral, and popliteal arteries in a segmental fashion, or it may cause diffuse involvement of these major arteries. The large arteries may be relatively unaffected with involvement chiefly limited to the terminal vessels, such as the anterior tibial, posterior tibial, and digital arteries and in rare instances even the arterioles. Frequently a combination of the various types of involvement is seen in the same patient. Although it remains predominantly a disease of the later decades of life, the incidence in individuals 40 to 50 years of age is increasing. Theories regarding the etiology implicate mechanical wear and tear associated with disturbances in cholesterol and lipid metabolism. Diet, heredity, occupation, endocrine imbalances, and local infection have variously been considered to play an important role in the general problem. Diabetes mellitus and hypertension are associated with an increased incidence of this disease. Males are predominantly affected in a ratio of 5 or 6 to 1.

Pathology

The lesions in middle aged patients are atheromas, which develop on the intimal surface of the vessels as small, yellow, elevated plaques that are composed of connective tissue cells and large quantities of lipoid material. These atheromatous plaques enlarge progressively, and fragmentation of the internal elastic membrane beneath the plaque follows. Irregular thinning and fragmentation of the muscle comprising the medial coat of the vessel occurs. Degeneration of the intimal surface promotes thrombus formation, which may undergo partial organization and recanalization. With cessation of blood flow to an area, necrosis or gangrene develops.

Symptoms and Signs

The symptoms of arteriosclerosis obliterans are due to tissue ischemia. Pain is the common symptom, and the severity and type of pain depend upon the degree of tissue ischemia. Usually the earliest symptom is intermittent claudication, an aching or cramp-like pain, which results from exercise and is quickly relieved by rest. This is most commonly noted in the calf but may also be appreciated in the foot or thigh. The distance that the patient is able to walk before developing pain is related to the degree of arterial occlusion. With progression of the disease there is decrease in the distance required to produce pain.

As more severe tissue ischemia develops, rest pain is appreciated in the digits and foot. This is described as a dull ache, which occurs most commonly at night. Local tissue involvement in the form of ulceration and gangrene is usually associated with local pain in the region of the lesion. When occlusion of the larger vessels occurs, such as the femoral or external iliac arteries, ischemic neuropathy is likely to develop. The pain of ischemic neuropathy is usually described as a constant, dull, numb sensation, which may be associated with paroxysmal electric shock-like stabs of pain in the distribution of the involved nerve. In addition to pain, joint stiffness, muscle weakness, paresthesias and sensory disturbances, and sensitivity to cold are usually present.

Examination invariably reveals impairment or absence of arterial pulsations to palpation. This is such an important and consistent physical finding that if the arterial pulsations are normal in the presence of lower extremity symptoms, one can rule out the possibility of arteriosclerosis obliterans.

Color changes of the feet, such as marked pallor or cyanosis, are not seen unless the degree of arterial occlusion is severe. However, abnormal pallor of the feet on elevation, slowly developing rubor, and delay in filling of superficial veins on dependency are signs of occlusive arterial disease that may be noted earlier in the course of the disease. The limb most affected by arteriosclerosis obliterans often has a lower skin temperature than the less affected side, and this difference may be gross enough to be obvious on simple palpation. Trophic changes, ulceration, and gangrene usually are noted first in the terminal portions of the digits as complications in advanced arteriosclerosis obliterans. Atrophy of the muscles, skin, and soft tissues is also a common finding in severe cases. If the disease progresses to a point requiring long periods of bed rest and avoidance of weight bearing, x-rays of the ankle and foot may reveal osteoporosis.

Arteriography and aortography are not advisable as routine diagnostic procedures, but they are of great importance if surgery is contemplated for removal of the arterial obstruction.

Treatment

Once this condition has been recognized clinically, there is a tendency for worsening to occur either in sporadic episodes or progressively with the passage of time. No treatment can rectify the organic arterial obstruction other than a surgical by-pass procedure utilizing an arterial graft, which proves to be of benefit in relatively few suitable cases. In spite of the ultimately poor general prognosis, particularly in elderly individuals in whom involvement of the extremities is often an indication of more widespread disease affecting the heart, brain, and other vital organs, active therapy may arrest the progress of the disease and afford symptomatic relief.

The general principles in the management of all occlusive arterial disease should be applied. Vasoconstricting influences, such as exposure to cold and the use of tobacco, should be avoided. The patient should be carefully instructed about proper foot care and the importance of preventing any local injury or infection that may lead to gangrene.

The value of the low cholesterol diet is uncertain, but if the patient is obese, a weight reducing diet is helpful if merely to lessen the trauma of weight bearing on ischemic feet. Long-term anticoagulant therepy is theoretically sound, but in practice its advantages have not been clear. The use of various drugs, including whiskey, to produce vasodilatation may be useful particularly in the milder cases.

If the obstructing arterial lesion is localized and arterial occlusive disease is not present distally, a by-pass procedure in which a direct surgical attack is made upon the obstructive lesion is the treatment of choice. This is accomplished by a variety of techniques. By-pass grafts utilizing the saphenous vein from the patient, a preserved femoral homograft, or a synthetic prosthesis have all been used with varying degrees of success. Excision of the arteriosclerotic plaque and obstructing thrombus by means of arteriotomy has also been carried out.

Sympathetic Block and Sympathectomy. The transient effect obtained by sympathetic block with local anesthetics is of no value in the managment of arteriosclerosis obliterans. It cannot be used as a criterion in the selection of suitable cases for sympathetic ganglionectomy because the desired persistent vasodilatation, which may lead to increased collateral circulation, cannot be achieved by a block.

The chief value of sympathectomy is in offering some protection against gangrene or ulceration in the event of local tissue injury. The increased blood flow to the muscles is minimal compared to the increased blood flow to the skin. For this reason, rest pain, which is often due to superficial tissue lesions, may be improved and minor ulcerative and gangrenous lesions may heal, but no improvement in the muscle symptoms of intermittent claudication will be realized following sympathectomy. The improved blood flow to the skin is thought by some to be the basis for the rare paradoxical effect of sympathectomy. This refers to increased ischemia of the digits following the operation that is due to a shunting of the circulating blood away from the distal portion of the extremity and to the more proximal portions of the skin.

Since lumbar sympathectomy can be performed with minimal risk and benefits approximately half of all patients with arteriosclerosis obliterans, the indications for the procedure are rather broad. Indications include patients who are not suitable for a by-pass procedure and also those who have had a blood vessel graft that subsequently has thrombosed. The only valid contraindication for this surgery is the patient whose general condition is so poor that any elective procedure is contraindicated because of the high risk involved.

When the likelihood of ultimate skin necrosis and infection is great or if rest pain is severe and the surgical risk is considered excessive, blocking of the sympathetic ganglia by the use of alcohol may be attempted.

Technique of Alcohol Block of Lumbar Sympathetic Ganglia. For a unilateral block the patient is placed in the lateral position with the legs and thighs flexed to obtain a maximal curve of the lumbar spine (Fig. 144). The side to be injected is uppermost. When a bilateral block is planned, the prone position is employed with the desired flexion of the lumbar spine obtained by placing several pillows under the abdomen. The interspace between the third and fourth lumbar vertebrae is identified as the first interspace above the level of the iliac crest.

A skin wheal is made 1½ inches to 2 inches lateral to the upper edge of the spinous processes of the second, third, and fourth lumbar vertebrae, the greater distance being used for larger individuals. A 20-gauge, 5-inch spinal needle with a depth marker is inserted through the wheals perpendicular to the longitudinal plane of the body but with a slight medial inclination (20 degrees). The needle is advanced until the point impinges upon the transverse process, usually at a depth just short of 2 inches. The depth marker is then placed 2 inches from the skin and the needle withdrawn until the point is in the subcutaneous tissue. The skin is then drawn about a quarter of an inch caudad and the needle directed more medially at an angle of 45 degrees with the sagittal plane. Advance of the needle will cause it to pass inferior to the transverse process and contact the lateral surface of the body of the vertebra.

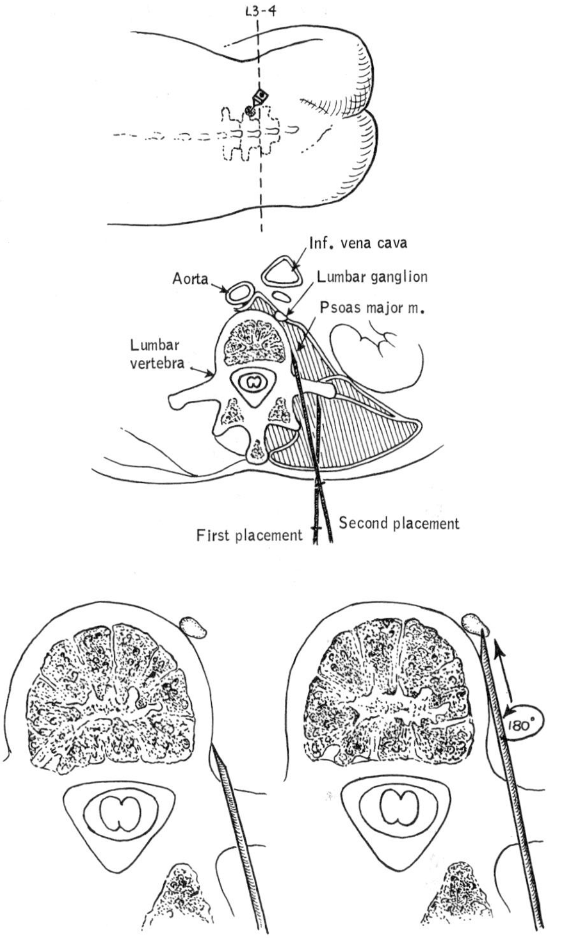

Figure 144. Alcohol block of lumbar sympathetic ganglion. The needle is best introduced with the bevel facing laterally, and when the vertebral body is contacted, a 180 degree rotation of the needle places the bevel adjacent to the bony surface, allowing it to glide over the body of the vertebra until the proper depth is reached.

The needle is best introduced with the bevel facing laterally, and when the vertebral body is contacted, a 180-degree rotation of the needle should allow the bevel to slide along the surface of the bone until the depth marker is flush with the skin. A proper placement of the needle results in the point's being located on the anterolateral surface of the vertebral body just anterior to the medial attachment of the psoas muscle. The stylet is withdrawn from the needle, and the procedure is repeated until all three needles are properly placed. To avoid inadvertent injection into the subarachnoid space or a blood vessel, aspiration is carefully performed before 3 cc. of 2 per cent procaine is injected through each needle. Rapid warming and drying of the lower leg and foot indicates a satisfactory sympathetic block and gives assurance of satisfactory position of the needles. Five cubic centimeters of 95 per cent alcohol is then injected slowly through each needle.

Control of Pain. The pain of intermittent claudication is a most difficult problem to treat. No drug exists that will effectively control this disabling symptom with any degree of dependable regularity. The use of deinsulinized pancreatic extract (Depropanex) may be effective occasionally in increasing the walking distance before intermittent claudication occurs. There is no well-supported explanation for this action, but one series of injections may be given a trial on an empiric basis. If improvement follows, this may be repeated. The usual course consists of one 2 cc. injection of Depropanex daily for one week, two injections weekly for the next four weeks, and one injection weekly for the next eight weeks.

Patients with intermittent claudication should be instructed that this is a protective warning symptom, and they should not attempt to continue walking after the pain develops because of the danger of injury to ischemic feet and toes.

If the patient is obese, weight reduction occasionally results in improvement of intermittent claudication by decreasing the work load of the muscles.

Rest pain may be due to ulceration and gangrene, ischemic neuropathy, or a combination of both. Sedatives, analgesics, and tranquilizers should be administered liberally. The administration of alcohol in the form of whiskey or brandy may be effective and useful in the treatment of rest pain.

The oscillating bed has been effective in the treatment of severe rest pain. By alternately raising and lowering the lower extremities above and below the level of the heart, this device presumably improves blood flow. The oscillations should be adjusted just short of pallor when the feet are up and just short of minimal rubor when they are down. Although it is of value in providing symptomatic relief from rest pain, it is questionable whether any permanent improvement in circulation results from the use of the ocillating bed. It is of no value for the treatment of intermittent claudication.

Some patients are so debilitated by severe rest pain that they present acute problems in management. They are admitted to the hospital in an exhausted state due to loss of sleep and with an inadequate food and fluid intake extending over a prolonged period of time. These patients commonly have protein deficiency and may be in electrolyte imbalance. If large amounts of opiates have been used to control their pain at home for a prolonged period of time, they may also have an addiction problem. Such extreme situations are best managed by providing continuous anesthesia of the lower extremities by means of an inlying epidural or caudal catheter. This gives the patient a needed respite during which he can rest comfortably and take adequate food and fluids. After three days the catheter is removed and routine measures instituted.

The crushing of sensory nerves of the lower extremity in an effort to achieve relief of the pain of gangrene and ulceration is of far less value in arteriosclerosis obliterans than in thromboangiitis obliterans. The healing of such surgical wounds is often poor, and they frequently break down owing to the generally inadequate circulation. The eventual prognosis of the two diseases is somewhat different, and this difference dictates a difference in approach with regard to pain management. Buerger's disease has a tendency to be self-limiting, and it is the hope that with persistent conservative treatment an adequate collateral arterial anastomosis will develop to carry blood around the occluded arterial segments. This is the mechanism by which many patients with Buerger's disease who have had ulceration and gangrene have eventually been restored to useful function with only minor residual symptoms. Arteriosclerosis obliterans, on the other hand, is characterized by a tendency for progressive worsening. For this reason intractable pain in this disease that cannot be controlled by adequate medical treatment may be considered an indication for amputation even if gangrene is not present.

chapter nine —

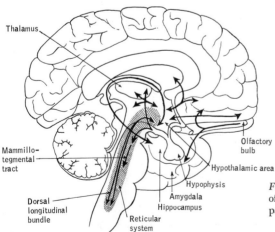

Figure 145. Diagrammatic representation of neuronal circuits related to the persistent pain of reflex dystrophies.

Reflex Dystrophies

The painful conditions included in this chapter have widely differing etiologies and would seem to be unrelated. However, critical analysis of these disorders demonstrates a striking similarity of clinical features as well as underlying pathophysiologic mechanisms in spite of the varying etiologic factors. The three major reflex dystrophies are causalgia, phantom limb pain, and central pain. The pain of all these conditions is usually constant and somewhat diffuse by comparison with the segmental or peripheral nerve distribution of neuralgia. Hyperesthesia is frequently associated with the pain. In all these conditions a reflex disorder is established, which to some extent involves the sympathetic nervous system. The exacerbation of pain by central phenomena, such as visual and auditory stimuli and emotional stress, is characteristic.

The persistent pain of causalgia, phantom limb, and thalamic pain is probably dependent upon neuronal circuits between the thalamus and cortex that maintain a sustained state of excitation even when the peripheral impulses that ordinarily induce pain have been cut off. The reticular activating system located in the brain stem may be related to this problem in a manner that has yet to be understood. The anatomic responses may be activated by the rhinencephalon and limbic systems through hypothalamic connections whose reverberating circuits connect with the neocortex (Fig. 145).

CAUSALGIA

Causalgia is a pain syndrome that follows injury to a peripheral nerve. It is characterized by burning pain, which is spontaneous, persistent, diffuse, and often severe and which is aggravated by emotional stimuli, touch, or motion. The pain is generally associated with vasomotor and dystrophic changes and, if prolonged, tends to create profound changes in the emotional state of the patient. There are a number of related conditions that are manifested by vasomotor or dystrophic disturbances with pain playing a less important role. These may be classified as "minor causalgias" and have been given a variety of names, each of which stresses different aspects of the disorder, such as "reflex dystrophy of the extremities," "Sudeck's atrophy," "trophic edema," "post-traumatic painful osteoporosis," "reflex arterial spasm," and many others.

Causalgia is a fairly common military medical problem owing to the large numbers of injured extremities occurring during war. However, improved techniques in management of long bone fractures and repair of major blood vessels have resulted in preservation of severely injured extremities, which some years ago would have been amputated. These advances have resulted in an increased incidence of causalgia in civilian life.

Severe, persistent, diffuse pain following nerve injuries was recognized by many early physicians. Ambroïse Paré treated King Charles IX of France for a causalgia-like pain resulting from a lancet wound of the extremity performed to induce bleeding for the treatment of a fever. It remained, however, for Weir Mitchell and his associates to give an account of the disease, which is so lucid that it stands today as a monumental classic of clinical description. His observations were made during the Civil War on Union soldiers treated at the Turner's Lane Hospital for Nervous Diseases in Philadelphia. In a subsequent book he first presented the term causalgia, which was quickly and universally accepted.

Signs and Symptoms

The onset of pain varies from immediately after the injury to an interval of several weeks later. The pain is typically constant, intense, diffuse, and burning. Terms such as aching, throbbing, stinging, or "pins and needles" may also be used to describe the pain, but direct questioning usually reveals a burning quality to the pain. In severe cases the pain is not limited to the sensory distribution of the injured nerve but extends well beyond its confines and is most severe in the peripheral portion of the affected limb.

There are often two distinct types of pain. Burning pain is appreciated in the skin, palm, finger tips, sole of the foot, and toes. Aching pain predominates deep in the tissues. The pain may be limited to the territory of the injured nerve in milder cases, or sometimes early symptoms of causalgia remain within the nerve boundaries, but as the disease becomes progressively more severe, the pain becomes more diffuse and involves the entire extremity. The skin of the area is hyperalgesic, particularly in the digits, palm of the hand, and sole of the foot.

The affected joints are often maintained rigidly to prevent severe pain produced by movement. In addition to movement, paroxysms of excruciating pain may be set off by almost any stimulus. Contact with clothing, drafts of air, noises, emotional stress, and eating or drinking may all aggravate the pain. Any precipitous change in temperature, either warm or cold, may increase the pain. Many patients derive partial relief from wet applications and constantly keep the part enveloped in wet cloth. Although most prefer a wet, cool environment, a significant number realize some relief with warm, wet soaks. If the pain is prolonged, the patient develops into a nervous recluse who adopts such elaborate precautions to prevent paroxysms of pain that they may seem absurd. Apathy associated with a haggard and woebegone expression reflecting constant, severe suffering is the typical picture of this disease.

These patients may be difficult to examine because of their fear of any disagreeable stimulus. Any attempt to perform the usual detailed sensory examination using a pin in an effort to determine the area of sensory defect almost invariably results in a clash between the physician and the patient. The use of a wisp of cotton may be tolerated, although many patients refuse to be subjected even to this minimal stimulus. The hyperalgesic skin is usually cool, mottled red, or cyanotic and dripping with perspiration. Less often the skin of the involved member is warm, dry, and scaly. After several weeks, the texture of the skin undergoes trophic changes and becomes shiny and glossy smooth. The nails become brittle and curved and the fingers tapering. In severe and protracted cases, x-rays reveal spotty areas of decalcification in the small bones of the hands or feet, which may continue on to more diffuse atrophic changes.

Pathophysiology

Causalgia is usually a complication of an incomplete peripheral nerve lesion. The median and sciatic nerves and the brachial plexus are most often involved. In addition to peripheral nerve damage, a variety of injuries to an extremity may rarely precipitate causalgia. Arterial and venous occlusions, amputations, fractures, and even sprains and trivial bruises have been reported as initiating the syndrome.

It is important, however, to understand the difference between neuralgia following damage to a major nerve and causalgia. Neuralgia is a frequent complication of a large variety of extremity injuries and is characterized by tingling or throbbing but not burning pain. The pain of neuralgia is usually restricted to the field of the affected nerve and, although uncomfortable, is not so severe as the pain of causalgia. High velocity, penetrating wounds are the most frequent cause of causalgia.

The route of transmission of the pain remains obscure, but there is little doubt that the sympathetic nerves play an important role in pain production. At the site of nerve injury a shunting of efferent sympathetic impulses into sensory fibers is thought to occur by some. Other theories relate to the influence of the sympathetics upon the blood vessels. Afferent impulses may be carried by sympathetic fibers along the major arteries, or peripheral vasospasm initiated by efferent vasoconstrictor impulses may produce hypoxemia, which in turn may irritate sensory nerve endings.

Management

Untreated causalgia may subside spontaneously and within a period of time varying from months to years may disappear completely. This is not the usual

211

natural course of the disease, however, and unless proper treatment is instituted, progressive worsening is likely to occur. The symptoms may increase in intensity and area of involvement, the intractable pain leading eventually to drug addiction, invalidism, and even suicide.

Interruption of the sympathetic chain supplying the painful part is the treatment of choice. The effects of sympathetic blocks utilizing local anesthetics are so constant in relieving or markedly alleviating pain that this procedure can be used as a diagnostic criterion of causalgia. A number of reports indicate that these blocks may have a therapeutic value, successive injections producing effects of greater duration until the symptoms either disappear entirely or become so mild that they no longer present a major problem. My personal experience has not borne out the therapeutic effectiveness of local anesthetic blocks. Although pain relief is accomplished when the sympathetic chain is infiltrated, the duration of relief is not prolonged beyond the effect of the local anesthetic. This may be due in part to the length of time the disease has been present. Most of the patients I have treated have had the pain of causalgia for many weeks or months. It is possible that sympathetic blocks instituted early in the course of the disease would have produced a therapeutic effect.

Sympathetic Block. When performing a sympathetic block for pain involving the upper extremity, one can attempt a stellate ganglion block via the anterior approach using 15 cc. of solution and elevating the patient's head in the hope that the anesthetic will infiltrate downward and affect the upper thoracic sympathetic chain. Injecting the ganglia individually by the posterior approach is more time consuming but may be necessary if the anterior approach is not effective. This method is illustrated in Figure 124 (p. 164). When the pain involves the lower extremity, a lumbar sympathetic block involving L1 to L4 is performed.

Sympathectomy. If several procaine blocks do not provide periods of pain relief that persist longer than the effects of physiologic block, sympathectomy should be performed.

Upper Extremity. The procedure of choice is the dorsal preganglionic sympathectomy with excision of the first, second, and third dorsal ganglia. This procedure is described and illustrated in Chapter 7.

Lower Extremity. Lumbar sympathectomy with removal of the second and third lumbar ganglia is illustrated in Chapter 8.

Physiotherapy. Following relief of severe pain after sympathectomy, the patient is able to tolerate physiotherapy. Whirlpool baths, active and passive movement, and gentle massage all enhance and speed recovery.

PHANTOM LIMB PAIN

Following an amputation, most individuals retain an awareness of the amputated part. This awareness may occur after amputation of an ear, nose, breast, or penis but is most commonly noted with loss of an extremity. The phenomenon was described by Amboïse Paré in 1551, but the term "phantom limb" was introduced more than 300 years later by S. Weir Mitchell.

Awareness of the phantom part usually occurs within the first several days following amputation. Initially it is experienced as a sensation of having the normal size and shape of the missing limb, but with the passage of time it tends to shrink and after several years may disappear entirely. Occasionally the phantom limb may be anatomically incomplete with only the ankle and foot appreciated or more rarely the knee and foot with no awareness of the intervening thigh and leg. Movement of the stump is often associated with an illusion of a corresponding movement of the phantom, and it is not unusual for the patient to have the impression of being able to move the phantom part voluntarily.

To some amputees the phantom limb is as real as the opposite intact extremity, and often the patient absent-mindedly attempts to use it. One of my patients was struck in the face by a tennis ball while watching a tennis match when he attempted to ward off a misdirected ball with his phantom upper extremity. Another patient was awakened from an afternoon nap by the telephone and forgetting that his lower extremity was missing, attempted to walk on the phantom. The use of an artificial arm or leg often causes a distinct change in the phantom. It may disappear entirely or more rarely exactly corresponds to the artificial limb.

Etiology

The exact mechanism causing the phantom phenomenon is not known. The various theories advanced to explain this phenomenon can be divided into two principal concepts: the peripheral irritation theory and the central nervous theory.

Peripheral Irritation Theory. Following any amputation, scar tissue formation occurs at the distal ends of the severed peripheral nerves. These end-bulb neuromas are thought to produce constant stimulation of the neurofibrils within the neuroma. Such a source of peripheral irritation is thought to give rise to impulses, which on reaching the thalamus form a self-perpetuating circuit between the thalamus and the cerebral cortex. This theory gave impetus to the performance of multiple procedures involving the stump in an effort to alleviate the occasionally painful phantom limb. Multiple reamputations at successively higher levels, excision of neuromas, revisions of the stump, and injections of the severed nerves and their neuromas with a variety of solutions were often performed in an effort to alter the phantom or provide relief of pain. Although relief of pain occasionally follows a local procedure upon the stump, the generally poor results have been used by its critics to refute the peripheral theory. The peripheral theory is also criticized because the phantom sensation does not follow a peripheral nerve distribution. I have treated several amputees with herniated lumbar discs associated with typical radiculitis down the phantom limb. With removal of the disc, the radiating pain ceased but the phantom was otherwise unchanged.

The Central Nervous Theory. Rather than considering peripheral irritation as the prime factor in producing the phantom, it is felt that this phenomenon is more likely related to facilitation due to central excitatory states at the highest integrative levels. At these integrative levels, both physiologic and psychic mechanisms are interrelated. From a psychologic standpoint, the gestalt theory or gestaltism, which is the tendency to perceive objects as a whole or complete unit, can be applied to the phantom limb phenomenon. Many examples of gestaltism are encountered in neurology. An individual with a homonomous hemianopsia who gazes directly into a mirror usually states that he sees an intact image of himself instead of only half an image. If a half circle is placed before this patient with the missing half of the circle toward the visual field cut, he will report the half circle as a full circle. Those who advance the gestalt theory consider the phantom limb as the patient's persisting concept of his total body image following the psychologic trauma related to the loss of a limb.

There is also a neurophysiologic basis for the total body image concept. Through multiple sensory impressions relayed to the sensory cerebral cortex and its association centers, the foundation of the body image is laid in infancy as the child becomes increasingly aware of the various parts of the body. The end-product of this sensory experience is the individual's developed image of himself, namely, his body image. In spite of anatomic changes, such as would occur from amputation of a limb, this body image is physiologically resistant to change. This resistance is thought to be the basis for the phantom phenomenon. Favoring this concept is the lack of phantom limbs in patients who were born with a missing limb or those who underwent amputation prior to the age of five years, before the body image was firmly established. The interesting observation was made that outcasts of society, such as derelicts from New York City's Bowery, rarely experience a phantom limb following amputation. This is thought to represent a gradual disintegration of the personality, which is associated with a progressive dissolution of the body image.

Paralysis of an extremity involving loss of sensation and motor power is frequently associated with the phantom phenomenon. The paralysis may be in the form of paraplegia due to spinal cord damage, hemiplegia from cerebral involvement, or peripheral nerve involvement, such as would occur from a brachial plexus lesion. In such cases, the phantom limb usually assumes a different position from the real but paralyzed limb or limbs. Paraplegics may report the sensation of having their paralyzed lower limbs drawn up in a tightly flexed knee-chest position when they are actually lying in flaccid extension. They frequently describe a feeling of having two pairs of legs. Since no amputation stump exists in these cases, this is another argument against the peripheral irritation theory.

Painful Phantom Limb

A variety of sensations may be appreciated in the phantom limb. Itching in the palm of the hand or sole of the foot is not unusual. Tingling, pins and needles, and mild pressure sensations are also rather common. Sometimes an unyielding rigidity may produce discomfort when the amputee is desperate to uncurl his missing toes or unclench his missing fist. Excitement, sickness, and weather changes may precipitate these sensations, which are often of moderate severity and can be tolerated by the patient. Occasionally these paresthesias assume an intensity that is intolerable, presenting a problem in management. Generally those phantoms that present a serious pain problem are painful within the immediate postamputation period, but it is not unusual for a painless phantom to eventually become painful.

The quality and intensity of the pain may vary from day to day in the same individual. The most common and persistent pain is a throbbing, burning sensation, which is usually felt most intensely in the foot or hand. Another common pain is appreciated as a cramped and twisted abnormal posturing of the limb, which is maintained immovably rigid in spite of the desire of the patient to change position. This latter type of pain does not occur when the patient has the illusion of being able to move the phantom voluntarily. The fist may be clenched tightly with the nails tearing into the palm. The pain may also be described as viselike, boring, and stabbing. Although the quality of the pain varies considerably, it is usually constantly present to some degree, exacerbation being precipitated by emotional stress, fatigue, and a variety of other stimuli.

Stump Pain

Although stump pain is often associated with phantom limb pain, the two conditions are not necessarily interrelated. It is possible for a patient to have a well-constructed painless stump in conjunction with a painful phantom, although it is more common to find some discomfort in the stump when the phantom is a source of serious pain. The stump pain may be characteristic of nerve compression neuralgia with a locally irritable end-bulb neuroma. In such instances the pain is usually localized in some portion of the amputation scar with hyperesthesia in this area. Any stimulation of this hypersensitive spot may cause sharp pain in the stump and occasionally radiating pains into the phantom limb. Occasionally the entire stump is hypersensitive to any manipulation, including light touch. The untreated, locally painful end-bulb neuroma may eventually progress to a more diffuse, severely painful hyperesthesia. Sometimes this diffuse pain is described as burning and is associated with vasomotor and sudomotor disturbances closely resembling causalgia.

Occasionally abnormal muscle activity is seen in the stump. This may be in the form of fibrillary twitching of small muscle bundles, or the entire stump may jerk involuntarily and spasmodically. This muscle activity is often precipitated by emotional stress, and I have seen patients who were apprehensive about undergoing what they feared would be a painful examination who found it necessary to maintain a constant and firm grip on the stump to prevent involuntary jerking movements.

Treatment

The management of phantom limb pain remains a difficult and frustrating problem, for no single method of therapy is uniformly successful. Entering into the complexity of the condition is the progressively changing nature

215

of the physiopsychologic mechanisms giving rise to the pain. It appears likely that in the early stages of this condition peripheral factors are predominant in the production of the pain. With the passage of time the seat of the dysfunction appears to progress to a more proximal site.

This impression appears to be supported by the occasional success of local procedures upon the stump in modifying and relieving phantom pain in the early stages of the disease. Anterolateral cordotomy is also of benefit in alleviating pain before the condition has become chronic and the cerebral cortex has become predominantly involved in projections of the painful phantom. No peripheral procedure is effective when cephalization of pain has occurred. This progressive centralization of the pain process makes inadvisable a prolonged period of deliberate inaction on the part of the physician in the hope that the discomfort will subside spontaneously. On the other hand any operative procedure that does not result in improvement worsens the situation from several points of view. Not only does valuable time elapse, but the discouragement of the patient invariably increases the difficulty of subsequent treatment. Any procedure that is planned must be based on a sound understanding of the problem and performed only after the most careful deliberation.

Treatment of the Stump. Most of these problems in civilian practice are managed initially by the general surgeon who performed the amputation. In my experience this management is usually excellent and reflects a proper appreciation of the complexities involved. Occasionally, however, patients with phantom limb pain are subjected to a series of ineffective surgical procedures including repeated resections of neuromas, multiple revisions of the stump, and reamputation at a higher level. Treatment of this nature flies in the face of all recorded experience with this problem, starting with S. Weir Mitchell's publications in 1871 to the present day.

Revision of the Stump. Reamputation at a higher level should never be considered for the relief of pain, since the pain invariably recurs in the new stump. The one justification for this procedure is a stump so badly constructed that fitting an artificial limb to it would not be feasible. If such is the case, a revision should be performed as soon as possible.

Painful Neuroma in the Stump. Point tenderness in the stump or an adherent, painful scar may be associated with a painful phantom. If the area of dysesthesia is localized, local infiltrations with procaine should be attempted. Progressively increasing periods of pain relief are thought by some to be an indication for a series of infiltrations in the hope of producing permanent relief. My experience with this form of therapy has not been encouraging, but those who claim favorable results emphasize initiating the infiltrations in the early stages of the disease. Since most of the patients I see for painful phantom have had the condition for prolonged periods of time, I may not be in a position to evaluate this method fairly.

Mechanical percussion of sensitive amputation neuromata has been employed in the past ten years for phantom limb pain associated with a locally painful area within the stump. This original and somewhat unique method of treatment was developed by Dr. Ritchie Russell after observing a patient with a painful digital amputation neuroma who was able to relieve his pain by striking the sensitive region repeatedly and vigorously against a solid object. When the painful neuroma is in the lower extremity, it is necessary to place one end of a wooden peg about an inch in diameter over the sensitive area and strike the other end rapidly with a wooden mallet for 10 to 20 minutes. The use of a mechanical vibrator over the painful area is another method of achieving the same result. Initially, percussion is performed several times daily, but with improvement in symptoms the duration and frequency of percussion can be reduced. Patients who obtain temporary relief from local injection of procaine are most likely to benefit from percussion. It is thought that the continued trauma produces progressive fibrosis of the nerve end with shrinkage of the neuroma.

When repeated infiltrations and mechanical percussion fail and if the pain is localized and can be relieved consistently by procaine infiltration, a single attempt at resecting the painful neuroma should be considered. The obvious problem is avoidance of neuroma reformation, which is accompanied by recurrence of pain within several weeks. Twenty per cent formalin, a 1 per cent aqueous solution of gentian violet injected into the freshly cut end of the nerve, or a 10 per cent solution of methyl methacrylate painted on the end of the cut nerve have all been used to prevent neuroma formation. After chemical fixation of the freshly cut nerve end with one of these solutions, the nerve end is then encased or capped with a snugly fitted sheath of some material that does not produce local tissue irritation, such as tantalum or polyethylene.

Sympathetic Block and Sympathectomy. Occasionally phantom limb pain is associated with vasomotor and sudomotor disturbances in the amputation stump. The stump may be cold, cyanotic, and hyperesthetic and during periods of discomfort may be covered with excessive quantities of perspiration. The pain is frequently increased by exposure to cold and emotional stress. A sympathetic ganglion block that will denervate the sympathetic outflow to the affected extremity is indicated in such a situation. This may cause a painful cold stump to become warm, dry, and nontender. Such a dramatic change is, of course, an indication for sympathectomy. Although it is reassuring to note a favorable change with sympathetic block prior to consideration of sympathetic surgery, one cannot rely entirely on the block as an infallible prognostic test. If the clinical signs and symptoms of vasomotor and sudomotor disturbance are present and the stump pain is of a burning quality, I would be in favor of sympathectomy despite equivocal results with a block.

Anterolateral Cordotomy and Rhizotomy. When a painful phantom limb is severe enough to incapacitate a patient and the previously described procedures are not indicated or have been unsuccessful, anterolateral cordotomy is the procedure of choice. There is a natural and reasonable reluctance to consider spinal cord surgery, which conceivably may result in unfortunate complications, such as sphincter impairment or paresis of the uninvolved extremity. Once a considered opinion has been reached that this operation is indicated, it is a mistake to defer action, since a prolonged period of suffering may lead to narcotic addiction and severe psychic disturbances. In addition, the progressive central displacement of the dysfunction may result in cephalization of the pain impulses once the condition becomes chronic.

217

This procedure presents no problem when the lower extremity is involved. The average level of analgesia varies from the costal margin to the umbilicus, and even taking into account the occasional fall in the initial level, it usually remains adequate. When the procedure is performed for pain in the upper extremity, certain technical difficulties arise and relief of pain is much more difficult to achieve. To obtain an adequate level of analgesia, it is necessary to incise the cord in the high cervical region, which carries greater risk than the usual upper thoracic anterolateral cordotomy. After an adequate level has been achieved with relief of the original pain in the upper extremity, a fall may result in the initial level of analgesia with recurrence of symptoms. If the level of the cordotomy is adequate, the local pain and tenderness within the stump itself are usually relieved. The likelihood that cordotomy will produce relief of painful phantom pain is not so great as in the case of a painful stump, but cordotomy remains the best neurosurgical procedure available. Because of the high level operation required to achieve relief of pain in the upper extremity, a large number of these patients are not helped by this procedure.

The problem of phantom limb pain in the upper extremity, which cannot be controlled adequately with cordotomy, has lead to the performance of a number of posterior rhizotomies in which the sensory roots innervating the painful extremity are cut. The complete loss of sensation that results from such an extensive sectioning of the posterior roots makes the deafferentated stump completely useless from a functional standpoint. Not only is this complete absence of sensation a source of annoyance to the patient, but it does not relieve the original phantom pain. For this reason the procedure should not be performed, since it only serves to worsen an already serious problem.

Resection of the Sensory Cortex. If carried to its logical conclusion, the theory involving the progressive migration of phantom limb pain cephalad, the pain eventually being projected by the cerebral cortex, would make resection of the sensory cortex a specific procedure for this condition. As far back as 1911, in a paper discussing sensory disturbances from cerebral lesions, Head and Holmes cited a case in which the phantom limb disappeared following a cerebrovascular lesion of the opposite parietal cortex. Further corroboration of this theory was supplied by reports describing the disappearance of painful phantoms following metastatic spread of cancer to the opposite parietal cortex and destruction of that area by a self-inflicted wound.

The operation involves the performance of a craniotomy under local anesthesia so that a complete mapping of the sensory representation of the affected limb can be carried out. After this area is mapped out, a cortical resection is carried out. When the procedure was introduced by Dr. de Gutierrez-Mahoney in 1944, the immediate results were encouraging. Unfortunately, long-term follow-up reports on patients subjected to sensory cortex resection indicate that the majority have recurrence of symptoms. It is felt that the reason for the large number of poor end-results is the wide extent of the sensory representation, behind the postcentral gyrus as well as within and in front of the precentral motor area, which is not well demonstrated on cortical stimulation. A frequent complication of this procedure, which involves operative trauma and subsequent scarring immediately adjacent to the motor strip, is epilepsy. In view of the predominantly poor long-term results of this procedure, it should not be considered as standard treatment for phantom limb.

Frontal Lobe Surgery. Several differing techniques and modifications of the original prefrontal lobotomy have been developed, all of them involving destruction of some portion of the frontal lobe, usually the frontal white matter. The purpose of such surgery is to suppress awareness of suffering and to diminish the reactive expression of pain. Unfortunately some mental deterioration is associated with damage of the frontal lobes sufficient to alter appreciation of pain. The various modifications in technique were devised mainly in the hope of producing pain relief with minimal psychologic changes. Selectivity in interrupting tracts or in removing limited areas of cerebrum has not revealed any one area in the frontal lobe that is specific with regard to pain control.

The severe psychologic deterioration that follows bilateral destruction of the frontal lobes is the major problem in this surgery. Dr. John E. Scarff extensively evaluated the advantages of unilateral frontal leucotomy in the hope that this modification would provide pain relief without severe psychologic deficit. Although the initial results of the procedure were promising, the pain returned in six or seven months in the majority of cases. Any frontal lobe surgery that is capable of providing relief of intractable pain for an indefinite period of time must be associated with disabling psychologic disturbances, and if psychologic recovery occurs, this is accompanied by a return of pain. Whenever this procedure is contemplated for intractable pain that is compatible with a normal life span, the emotional factor must be discussed completely with the family. They should be made aware that there is every likelihood of the patient's never being able to assume gainful employment. The care of these patients rests ultimately with the family, and unless they are completely prepared to assume responsibility for prolonged custodial and nursing care, it is ill advised to proceed with surgery of this nature.

Psychotherapy. If early psychologic supportive therapy is properly instituted, the chronically intractable, painful phantom limb that defies all therapy may never develop. When an elective amputation of a limb is planned, the physician should initiate a program of psychologic support in the preoperative period. Loss of a limb is invariably a severe emotional trauma to the patient not only because of the resulting functional handicap but because the fear of losing forever a long familiar part of the body is deeply painful. Expressions such as "a part of me is dying" reflect the sense of mourning over this limb. In this connection, many patients are squeamish about discussing the disposition of the amputated limb but may be apprehensive about the part's being handled disrespectfully. A tactful discussion regarding these and other problems is beneficial. If a severe depression follows the amputation, psychiatric help should be obtained. As soon as possible after the amputation, restoration of function should be instituted as vigorously as possible. In many instances, a prosthesis that is able to carry out some of the functions of the missing limb alleviates the pain. Many individuals are loath to discuss the phantom sensation with anyone for fear they will be labeled psychotic or neurotic. A brief discussion regarding this problem often allays their fears in this regard and is a beneficial factor in their phantom limb pain.

CENTRAL PAIN

The term "central pain" refers to pain that is directly or primarily produced by a lesion affecting the pain pathways within the central nervous system. Indirect or secondary pain related to central lesions, such as headache associated with the increased intracranial pressure caused by a brain tumor, does not fall into this classification. However, if the same tumor were to infiltrate the lateral nucleus of the thalamus and produce a burning pain affecting the side of the body opposite the lesion, this would be an example of central pain.

The lesion producing "central pain" may involve the spinothalamic tract at any level from the cord to the thalamus as well as the thalamocortical radiations from the thalamus to the cerebral cortex.

Mechanism of Central Pain

The mechanism of this phenomenon is not known, although several theories have been advanced. It was originally believed that the abnormal pain resulting from central nervous system lesions was due to irritation at the site of the lesion. This concept was supported by evidence demonstrating that stimulation of the pain pathways in the spinal cord, brain stem, and cerebral cortex often elicited pain. The "irritation theory" was rejected by Head and Holmes, who advanced their belief that lesions of the cerebral cortex affected certain corticothalamic inhibitory influences and that release of the thalamus from the inhibitory control of the cortex was responsible for central pain. Some believe that both "irritation" and reduction of central inhibition play a role in central pain. Adding to the difficulties in understanding and investigating central pain is its comparative rarity and unpredictability. Comparable lesions of the central nervous system may produce similar symptoms that would clinically indicate that they are in all respects identical, yet some are associated with central pain and others are pain-free.

The aggravation of this type of pain by psychic stress is so constant a factor that it can be assumed that regardless of the specific mechanism the pain is in some way connected in the highest integrative levels to circuits relating to the emotions. This combination of psychic and autonomic interrelationships may implicate the rhinencephalon and limbic systems, which activate autonomic impulses by means of connections with the hypothalamus.

Characteristics of Central Pain

Central pain is spontaneous, for it occurs in the absence of the usual extrinsic stimuli that ordinarily produce pain. Although it is generally persistent and constantly present, the severity of the pain varies considerably at different times. The quality of the pain is described in such terms as aching, gnawing, boring, burning, cold, and very frequently as a generally uncomfortable and unpleasant sensation, which the patient is unable to describe. Aggravation of the pain may occur spontaneously for no apparent reason, but the intensity may be increased by specific stimuli, such as anxiety, emotional stress, and sudden changes in temperature. Commonly there is an overreaction to stimuli that normally would not be considered painful so that touch, heat, cold, and pinprick may all cause a similar widespread, disagreeable sensation on the affected side while the same stimulus causes no discomfort on the normal side of the body. However, despite this overreaction to stimuli, the actual threshold for appreciation of a pinprick is often elevated. When this elevated pain threshold is reached by a pinprick, the pain may not necessarily be appreciated at the spot stimulated but may extend over a relatively wide area. Frequently there is an abnormally prolonged time lag between the onset of the painful stimulus and the appreciation of pain, which may then long outlast the stimulus. Often associated with the pain are signs of autonomic dysfunction, such as cyanosis, decrease in skin temperature, and increased sweating.

Spinal Cord Lesions with Central Pain

The most common cause of pain associated with spinal cord lesions is mechanical compression of posterior roots. Much more rarely, in various conditions affecting the spinal cord, pain is encountered that does not fall into the anatomic confines of the nerve root dermatomes and can only be explained on the basis of central pain. The typical diffuse, burning pain has been produced by stimulation of the spinal cord under local anesthesia. Syringomyelia may go through a stage in which there is involvement of the large sensory tracts of the spinal cord, which may be associated with remote pain ranging in severity from uncomfortable paresthesia to violent aching or burning pain. This pain is aggravated by direct stimulation, temperature changes, and psychic disturbances and is often an early symptom of the disease. With the passage of time it becomes associated with the classic form of sensory dissociation characterized by loss of pain and temperature sensation and preservation of touch. Spinal cord tumors may also cause central pain that is related to involvement of the spinothalamic fibers of the cord.

Trauma to the spinal cord, such as spinal concussion resulting from fracture dislocation, is an occasional cause of central pain resulting from a spinal cord lesion. Although the majority of pains from such trauma are related to nerve root compression at the site of the dislocation, one occasionally encounters pain that is remote from the site of involvement and can only be explained on the basis of central pain. This pain usually disappears within one or two weeks and is usually ignored, since it is often negligible in comparison with other symptoms. Although relatively few reports of this phenomenon have appeared, I believe this represents a lack of appreciation of the symptoms rather than a valid indication of its rarity.

Brain Stem Lesions with Central Pain

A small proportion of brain stem lesions produce pain, and when it occurs it is more common with lesions involving the medulla and pons rather than those involving the mesencephalon. This is because there are no sensory nuclei in the mesencephalon, while the descending sensory nucleus of the trigeminal nerve is located in the medulla and pons. The anatomy of the region may give rise to a crossed pain distribution, the face being affected on the side of the lesion and the trunk and limbs on the opposite side. This picture is the result of involvement of the descending nucleus of the trigeminal nerve, affecting the ipsilateral face, and the spinothalamic fibers, which cross to innervate the contralateral trunk and limbs. The quality of the pain is usually reported as aching or burning.

Thalamic Lesions with Central Pain

Thalamic lesions are the most commonly recognized cause of central pain. Although almost any lesion affecting the thalamus, such as tumor, inflammation, or trauma, may give rise to spontaneous pain, it is seen most often with vascular lesions of the thalamus, particularly lesions involving the lateral nucleus of this structure. The typical clinical picture was described extensively by Dejerine and Roussy in 1906, who first termed it the syndrome thalamique or thalamic syndrome. The components of the "thalamic syndrome" are as follows: (1) transient hemiparesis or hemiplagia due to temporary impairment of function without actual destruction of the adjacent internal capsule; (2) impairment of superficial and loss of deep sensation due to destruction in the thalamus of the terminations of the median lemniscus and spinothalamic tracts; (3) choreoathetoid movements, ataxia, and tremor due either to sensory defect or to involvement of the dentato-rubrothalamic tracts; and (4) spontaneous, intolerable pains and hyperpathia. All these symptoms and signs appear on the side opposite the lesion.

When the etiology of the thalamic syndrome is vascular, the posterior cerebral artery or its branches are involved. This vessel usually arises from the basilar artery but is sometimes a branch of the internal carotid artery. It conveys blood to the optic thalamus by means of the thalamogeniculate and thalamus-perforating branches and to the inferior and medial portions of the posterior temporal and occipital lobes, including the area striata. Thrombosis of the entire vessel or its branches determines the extent of the clinical picture, involvement of the smaller branches giving rise to a limited component of the thalamic syndrome. In extensive lesions the entire contralateral half of the body, including the head, may exhibit hyperpathic pain. In smaller lesions the pain is limited to large contiguous portions of the body, such as the entire lower extremity and lower portion of the trunk or the side of the head, upper extremity, and chest.

Characteristically, thalamic pains appear after an interval of several weeks as the patient is recovering from a thalamic infarct, although occasionally it is present with the onset of the disease. It varies in intensity from uncomfortable paresthesia to an intolerable aching, boring, or burning pain that is relatively unaffected by analgesics. It may be most severe in the distal portions of the extremities, and the patient may have the sensation that the hand or foot is being squeezed or twisted.

Hyperalgesia and hyperpathia are a part of the thalamic syndrome with excessive reaction to stimulation of the involved portions of the body. In addition to manifesting an overresponse to such cutaneous stimuli as stroking, deep pressure, and pinprick, temperature changes, particularly cold, and sudden noises or bright light may also aggravate the pain. When the patient is fatigued, debilitated from illness, or apprehensive, the pain is increased. The degree of sensory loss associated with the thalamic syndrome appears to have little or no relationship to the intensity of pain. Marked emotional lability with unmotivated crying or laughing is frequently manifested.

Lesions of the Cerebral Cortex with Central Pain

A number of cases have been reported with lesions involving the cerebral cortex and sparing the thalamus, manifesting central pain in the contralateral side of the body. Although many of these were cortical ischemic lesions resulting from cerebrovascular occlusive disease, a significant proportion were brain tumors and other mass lesions. This fact emphasizes the importance of a thorough neurologic evaluation prior to treating the patient for "thalamic pain" to avoid overlooking a possible surgical lesion.

Treatment

No treatment can be considered the solution to this rare but harassing problem. For pain that is most severe in the face, interruption of the trigeminal nerve by alcohol block or rhizotomy has been performed with a small percentage of successes. High cervical cordotomy has produced similarly disappointing results in cases of pain in the trunk and extremities. Sympathectomy is of no value in this condition. The only standard surgical procedure with even a reasonable likelihood of success is prefrontal lobotomy. This is best reserved for individuals who are so incapacitated from the neurologic deficit caused by the cerebrovascular disease that there is little hope of gainful function for the future. The use of tranquilizers may be helpful particularly in patients with a very marked emotional lability.

chapter ten –

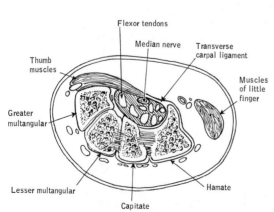

Figure 146. Anatomy of the carpal tunnel.

Nerve Compression Syndromes, Painful Scars, Postherpetic Neuralgia

The pain syndromes discussed in this section all result from trauma to peripheral nerves. The trauma may be in the form of pressure, transection of cutaneous nerves with subsequent neuroma formation, or the scarring and reaction following infection, as in postherpetic neuralgia.

MEDIAN NERVE COMPRESSION AT THE WRIST (CARPAL TUNNEL SYNDROME)

The median nerve is frequently subject to compression neuropathy at the wrist because of the anatomic relationships. As the nerve enters the carpal tunnel, it lies between the thick, unyielding transverse carpal ligament and the flexor tendons of the fingers (Fig. 146). Increased size of the tendons or ligaments, which might result from trauma or rheumatoid synovitis, and any alteration in the contour of the carpal tunnel resulting from bone deformity associated with osteoarthritis or fracture of the wrist bones could easily cause compression of the median nerve. The sensory distribution of this nerve is to the lateral half of the palm, the lateral half of the ring finger, and the palmar surface of the entire middle finger, index finger, and thumb (Fig. 147). The motor innervation of the nerve is to the opponens, short flexor, and short abductor muscles of the thumb.

Etiology

The carpal tunnel syndrome may result from several different causes.

225

Trauma to the wrist involving the distal end of the radius and the carpal bones is a relatively common cause. Any space-occupying mass within the carpal tunnel, such as tumor, ganglion, or tenosynovitis, will also compress the median nerve. Hypertrophy of the carpal bones from acromegaly and osteoarthritis are cited occasionally. A significant number of patients spontaneously develop compression neuropathy of the median nerve within the carpal tunnel without known cause. Spontaneous onset most often occurs in middle age. When, as is frequent, the condition occurs bilaterally, it is usually worse in the dominant hand, which would indicate that activity tends to aggravate the condition. Sometimes a specific activity brings on the symptoms, which subside with avoidance of the activity. I once examined a young college student who first noted these symptoms when he took a summer job that involved ladling out portions of food in a cafeteria. This not particularly strenuous activity required repeated hyperextension and hyperflexion of the wrist. His symptoms cleared when he stopped work to resume his classes in the fall. For some reason, women develop this condition more frequently than men in a ratio of about 3 to 1.

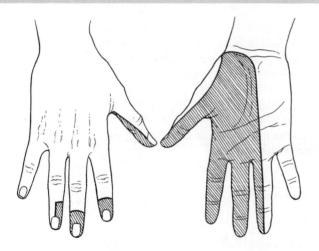

Figure 147. Sensory distribution of the median nerve.

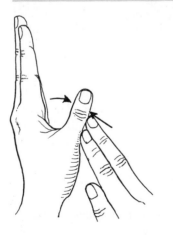

Figure 148. The strength of the short abductor and short flexor muscles to the thumb is tested by palmar abduction.

Signs and Symptoms

Pain, paresthesias, and subjective numbness within the sensory distribution of the median nerve in the hand are usually the first symptoms noted by the patient. Muscular weakness and atrophy in the thenar eminence with progressive weakness and clumsiness of the affected hand may sometimes progress to a surprisingly advanced state before the patient is aware of the motor disability. Pain commonly occurs at night and may reach a frequency and severity that seriously interferes with sleep for prolonged periods. Occasionally the aching and pain, in addition to involving the hand, radiate in a retrograde fashion up the forearm sometimes as high as the shoulder. In spite of extension of pain into the forearm and arm, sensory examination reveals hypesthesia confined to the hand.

Atrophy and weakness of the thenar muscles—opponens, short flexor, and short abductor muscles—is noted in long-standing cases. The strength of the short abductor and short flexor muscles to the thumb is tested by palmar abduction (Fig. 148). Occasionally the opponens pollicis muscle is spared despite thenar atrophy. The opponens can be tested by opposition of the thumb and little finger (Fig. 149). Maintenance of the wrist in hyperflexion or hyperextension for a minute is likely to precipate sensory symptoms. Gentle tapping on the volar surface of the wrist may produce a tingling sensation, which radiates into the sensory distribution of the median nerve in the hand.

The differential diagnosis includes cervical disc disease, spinal cord tumor, scalenus anticus syndrome, Raynaud's disease, syringomyelia, multiple sclerosis, and muscular dystrophy.

Treatment

The standard treatment for carpal tunnel syndrome is decompression of the median nerve by section of the transverse carpal ligament. Surgery is indicated when the symptoms are severe and of prolonged duration, when the sensory loss in the fingers and hand is progressive, or when muscle atrophy is noted. It is also indicated if, for economic reasons, a prolonged course of treatment that might not alleviate the condition would constitute a hardship, since the results of surgery are excellent while other methods involve a high rate of relapse. When the symptoms are mild and of short duration or the patient is opposed to surgery, two nonsurgical methods can be utilized.

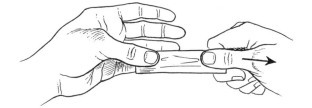

Figure 149. The opponens pollicis muscle can be tested by grasping a piece of paper between the thumb and little finger.

Immobilization. The use of an anterior splint extending from the upper portion of the forearm to the metacarpophalangeal joint in order to immobilize the wrist in a neutral position may be given a trial (Fig. 150). This splint is worn by the patient at night when the symptoms are usually most severe. If improvement is realized by this method, it usually is noted within three to six weeks. The incidence of recurrence of symptoms with this therapy is quite high.

Hydrocortisone Injection. Injection of hydrocortisone acetate suspension into the carpal tunnel often provides temporary relief, and occasionally the symptoms do not recur.

Technique of Injection. The tendons of the flexor carpi radialis and palmaris longus are identified by flexing the wrist against resistance (Fig. 151). The wrist is then maintained in moderate extension, and a procaine wheal is made just medial to the flexor carpi radialis tendon at the proximal crease of the wrist. A 25-gauge needle is introduced through the wheal, making a 70-degree angle with the forearm, and carefully advanced into the carpal tunnel. If resistance of the flexor finger tendons is encountered, rather than forcing the needle through the tendons, a path between them may be found by carefully moving the point of the needle from side to side. A dose of 25 mg. (0.5 cc.) of hydrocortisone is injected through the needle. For a day or two after the injection, the patient may appreciate increased discomfort, after which the symptoms subside.

Technique of Surgery. The procedure is best performed under general anesthesia, and although many use a pneumatic tourniquet to obtain a bloodless field, I prefer to control the bleeding as it occurs by using electro-

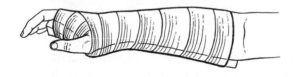

Figure 150. Anterior splint for immobilization of the wrist in a neutral position.

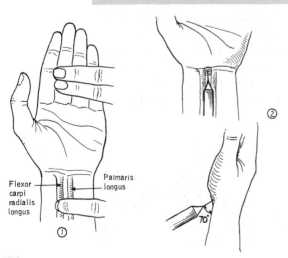

Figure 151. Technique of injecting hydrocortisone into the carpal tunnel. (1) Identification of the flexor carpi radialis and palmaris longus tendons. (2) Insertion of needle into carpal tunnel.

Flexor carpi radialis longus

Palmaris longus

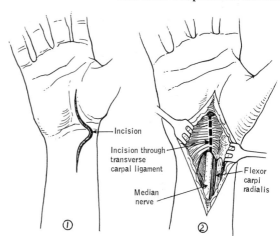

Figure 152. Technique of section of transverse carpal ligament. (1) Skin incision. (2) Line of incision through transverse carpal ligament.

Incision

Incision through transverse carpal ligament

Median nerve

Flexor carpi radialis

①

②

cautery. The incision starts on the volar surface of the forearm an inch and a half above the proximal flexion crease, curves laterally at the flexion crease, and sweeps medially to connect with the midpalmar crease (Fig. 152). A straight skin incision crossing the flexion crease of the wrist is to be avoided because of the possible complication of flexion contracture at the wrist if the scar goes on to keloid formation. The fascia in the forearm between the flexor carpi radialis and palmaris longus is divided, exposing the median nerve. The transverse carpal ligament is divided with a scissors, avoiding trauma to the underlying median nerve. Occasionally the nerve appears swollen beneath the transverse carpal ligament and a pressure neuroma can be seen, but in most cases the anatomy of the exposure is not grossly remarkable. Closure of the skin is performed using interrupted black silk technique in two layers. A seven- to ten-day period of postoperative disability involving the operated hand occurs so that it is unwise to perform surgery on both hands simultaneously when the condition is bilateral.

ULNAR NERVE COMPRESSION AT THE ELBOW

The ulnar nerve is given off from the brachial plexus in the axilla. It passes down the extremity medial to the brachial artery until it reaches the distal third of the arm, where it diverges from the brachial artery to enter the groove between the medial epicondyle of the humerus and the olecranon. The ulnar nerve passes between the humeral and ulnar heads of the flexor carpi ulnaris muscle and descends to the wrist and hand along the ulnar aspect of the forearm.

Etiology

Within this bony groove at the elbow, the nerve is susceptible to compression either from direct trauma to the elbow or from changes within the

229

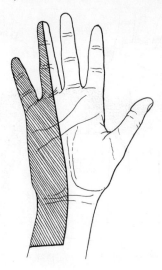

Figure 153. Sensory distribution of the ulnar nerve.

groove that cause gradual impingement upon the nerve. Sometimes a slowly progressive ulnar nerve palsy is the delayed result of a previous fracture or severe soft tissue injury about the elbow, leading to eventual scarring. Changes in configuration of the groove due to osteoarthritis are occasionally seen in conjunction with ulnar nerve damage. In addition to severe direct trauma to the elbow joint, which may produce immediate or delayed ulnar palsy, repeated mild trauma may also be an overlooked factor. Habitual leaning of the elbow upon a desk or table or constant use of the elbow as a support at work may cause a tardy ulnar palsy. I once treated a man who was employed as a riveter in an aircraft factory. His particular task necessitated using a small riveting machine while lying on his side, supported by his left elbow. The rapid vibration of the machine in association with the pressure upon the elbow caused a slowly progressive left ulnar palsy. The restricted opening through which the nerve passes at the elbow is formed by an aponeurotic arch between the olecranon and the medial epicondyle, the floor of this arch being the medial ligament of the elbow joint. This relatively unyielding passageway is somewhat snug so that extensive tissue edema in this region may produce nerve compression.

Signs and Symptoms

Sensory changes involving the ulnar aspect of the hand and wrist, including the ulnar side of the ring finger, are often the earliest signs of tardy ulnar palsy (Fig. 153). Associated with impairment of sensation is a variable degree of discomfort in this area in the form of tingling and aching. The pain is usually worse at night. One of the first motor signs in tardy ulnar palsy is the tendency of the little finger to drift away from the other digits and to take a position of slight flexion. With progression of the condition, atrophy and weakness occur in all muscles innervated by the ulnar nerve.

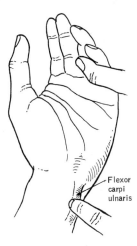

Figure 154. The flexor carpi ulnaris is tested by pressing on the palmar surface of the flexed little finger and palpating the tendon of the flexor carpi ulnaris.

Flexor
carpi
ulnaris

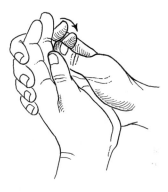

Figure 155. The medial half of the flexor digitorum profundus is tested by flexing the distal phalanges of the little and ring fingers against resistance.

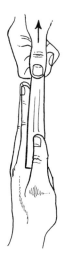

Figure 156. The adductor pollicis is tested by grasping a slip of paper between the thumb and radial border of the hand.

231

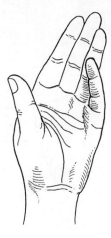

Figure 157. The opponens digiti quinti is tested by moving the extended little finger toward the radial side of the hand.

The *flexor carpi ulnaris* is tested by pressing on the palmar surface of the flexed little finger and palpating the tendon of the flexor carpi ulnaris (Fig. 154). The *flexor digitorum profundus* (medial half) is tested by flexing the distal phalanges of the little and ring fingers (Fig. 155). In testing the *adductor pollicis,* the patient resists attempted withdrawal of a piece of paper grasped between the thumb and the radial border of the hand (Fig. 156). The *opponens digiti quinti* is tested by moving the extended little finger toward the radial side of the hand (Fig. 157).

In addition to motor weakness, the spaces between the tendons on the dorsum of the hand, particularly the interval between the index finger and the thumb, are converted into hollows, indicating atrophy of the interossei, the third and fourth lumbricales, and the adductor pollicis. A flattening of the hypothenar eminence occurs because of atrophy of the palmaris brevis and muscles of the little finger. Tapping the area of the ulnar groove often produces radiation down the ulnar aspect of the forearm.

Treatment

The standard treatment for ulnar nerve compression at the elbow is transplantation of the ulnar nerve (Fig. 158). This is not a technically difficult procedure and the results are generally excellent.

An 8-inch incision is outlined along the medial aspect of the arm and forearm centering on the medial epicondyle. Rather than extend the incision directly over the bony prominence of the epicondyle, the middle of the incision is curved anteriorly. The upper portion of the incision is carried down to the brachial fascia, which is then opened carefully to avoid injury to the ulnar nerve, which lies just below it. The ulnar nerve is easily located posterior to the medial intermuscular septum in a longitudinal groove of the triceps muscle. After freeing up the normal portion of the nerve, the dissection is carried down into the elbow. The fascia overlying the nerve in the elbow must be carefully dissected free, since this is often an area of scarring

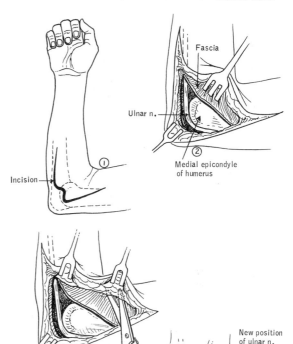

Figure 158. Technique of ulnar nerve transplant. (1) Skin incision. (2) The ulnar nerve is first exposed in the upper portion of the incision. (3) and (4) Preparation of a new bed for the ulnar nerve by dissecting a full thickness flap of skin laterally.

and the nerve may be quite adherent to the surrounding tissues. The nerve is then dissected free in the forearm by separating the fibers of the flexor carpi ulnaris. A full thickness flap of skin is dissected laterally. The nerve is transplanted to its new bed, and several black silk sutures may be used to tack down subcutaneous fat to the underlying fascia in order to prevent medial migration of the nerve.

Too short an incision may cause dissection of an insufficient length of nerve for transplantation, producing traction upon the nerve at either end of the dissection (Fig. 159). I must also caution against suturing the nerve into a bed of fascia, since this also may increase nerve compression.

PAINFUL SCARS

Cutaneous scars of wounds, surgery, or burns are occasionally a source of discomfort. The pain may vary from a mild localized tenderness or pressure to a continuous aching or burning dysesthesia, which extends beyond the im-

233

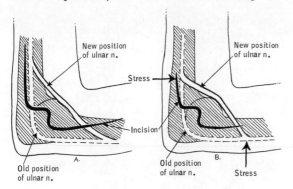

Figure 159. If too short a segment of nerve is dissected free, transplantation will produce traction upon the nerve at either end of the dissection.

mediate area of the scar. Cold, damp weather, pressure or manipulation of the scarred skin, and emotional factors may all aggravate the discomfort. If the scar extends over a considerable area, which is frequent with burn scars, reduced mobility of the involved area is often present because of the widespread cicatrices. In such instances, attempts to increase the range of mobility intensify the pain.

The appearance of the scar is often misleading; many well-approximated "hair line" incisions are a source of discomfort, and often a thick, indurated scar goes on to keloid formation and still remains quite painless. Scars in certain areas of the body are particularly prone to develop into pain problems. Herniorrhaphy scars are more apt to result in persistent aching pain than other abdominal incisions. A scar that is relatively fixed to bony prominences, as might occur in the anterior tibial area and the malleolar and condylar regions, is likely to remain troublesome. Injuries or operative procedures involving the thoracic cage often result in disabling intercostal neuralgia.

Pathology

Neuromas, either in continuity or as end-bulb neuromas developing from the severed ends of nerves, are the usual cause of painful scars. Microscopic examination of cutaneous scars reveals many tortuous, small nerve fibers, which are thicker than normal and nodular and terminate in little whorls; small neuromas are seen throughout. Organization of scar tissue may take months and even years, and the time that may elapse between wound healing and development of a painful scar also varies considerably.

Treatment

Precipitous action in the excision of painful scars is often the opening salvo of a long and fruitless siege, which might have been avoided by conservative therapy and a little patience. Thyroidectomy scars and other transverse neck incisions are often annoying, particularly to the nervous and apprehensive patient who complains of painful tugging and pulling and difficulty in swallowing. No experienced thyroid surgeon would consider early revision of a well-healed thyroidectomy scar on the basis of these symptoms. Any surgeon considering such a procedure should realize that further surgery must result in increased scar tissue. Reassurance and careful instruction in massage of the anterior cervical area will in time benefit the majority of these patients.

Painful abdominal scars are often extremely tender in one point. This is usually the site of a neuroma, and palpation, if tolerated by the patient, may reveal a nodule at the site of tenderness. If procaine infiltration of this tender nodule alleviates the pain, a series of at least six infiltrations should be given before considering excision of the scar. These injections are spaced at weekly intervals initially, and if the pain decreases, the interval is progressively increased. Attempts to relieve symptoms by cutting sensory nerves leading to the painful area are often encouraging initially, but long-term results are usually poor. This method is attempted frequently with painful herniorrhaphy scars, since procaine infiltration of the ilioinguinal and iliohypogastric nerves medial to the anterior spine of the ilium frequently produces prompt but temporary relief of pain. Surgical section of the nerves usually results in recurrence of the original pain within one or two months, which may be compounded by an unpleasant neuralgia from the severed nerves.

Intercostal neuralgia is often a disabling symptom following wounds or surgery of the thoracic cage. Here again resection of neuromas and proximal neurectomy have been disappointing. The use of a series of local anesthetic injections and patience is often the most rewarding approach. In some cases relief can be obtained by blocking the intercostal nerve proximal to the neuroma. If this is ineffective, it is necessary to resort to paravertebral blocks. A series of such infiltrations is frequently beneficial.

Surgery for Painful Scars. When an adequate period of conservative management has failed to provide relief of pain, a single local attack upon the scar or the painful neuroma is indicated. In view of the high percentage of failures from these procedures, the surgeon should explain the problem completely to the patient. A local procedure of this type is quite minor compared with the major procedures of rhizotomy or spinothalamic cordotomy, which should be considered only after local procedures have proved ineffective. Rhizotomy, in which the painful area is deafferentated by sectioning the necessary posterior roots, has a moderately successful chance of success. Its best application is for intercostal neuralgia, which usually has a segmental character approximating the nerve root dermatomas. Even with this type of lesion one cannot reasonably guarantee success. The only surgical procedure that can be considered "certain" is spinothalamic cordotomy. This, of course, is a major procedure and is considered when everything short of this surgery has failed.

POSTHERPETIC NEURALGIA

Herpes zoster (shingles) is an acute, self-limiting viral infection, which produces inflammatory lesions in the posterior root ganglia. The disease is characterized clinically by pain and a vesicular skin eruption in the distribution of the affected ganglia. An occasional complication of this disease is the persistence of severe intractable pain within the area of the original cutaneous eruption. This postherpetic neuralgia, which is seen chiefly in elderly patients, is one of the most annoying and tormenting pain syndromes. The unrelenting pain, causing sleepless nights and intolerable days, may be so intractable that patients are willing to undergo any treatment to obtain relief.

The cause of this condition is not understood. The inflammatory lesions may result in scarring and degenerative changes involving the spinal cord, ganglia, nerve trunks, and skin, and this may be a factor in persistent postherpetic pain. The disease occurs primarily in the ganglia of the spinal cord, but occasionally the cranial nerves are involved.

Treatment

The results of treatment are not good and often the postherpetic pain is intractable to all forms of therapy.

Analgesic Blocks. Although an occasional "cure" is reported following nerve root block with local anesthetic, my experience with this method has been uniformly poor.

Deep x-ray therapy of the affected ganglia has been recommended by some with variable results.

Section of sensory nerve roots (cranial or spinal, depending on the site of pain) has occasionally resulted in improvement. Most patients continue to have pain in spite of extensive rhizotomies, which cause complete numbness in the painful regions.

Spinothalamic Cordotomy. When the pain is below the costal margin and the sensory level produced by cordotomy is well above the pain, a significant number of patients will be relieved. Even with this procedure, however, there are several reports of more than adequate sensory levels with persistence of pain.

Excision of wide segments of involved skin has been performed with occasional encouraging results in several cases. The lesion must be in the abdomen or thoracic region for this method of therapy to be used.

Prefrontal Lobotomy. When every available treatment has been given a trial and has failed, prefrontal lobotomy is occasionally considered. In my opinion, the price that must be paid in the great sacrifice of personality and mentation is so great that this procedure is justified only in very special circumstances, if ever.

chapter eleven

Intractable Pain and Cancer

chapter eleven —

Intractable Pain
and Cancer

Pain of malignant disease varies in intensity, but it rarely, if ever, reaches the severity of renal colic, tic douloureux, or the other excruciating pains encountered in medical practice. It is the chronic and prolonged duration of this intractable discomfort, over a period of weeks and months, that in time erodes the endurance of even the most resolute to create one of the most difficult problems in pain management. The relentless downhill course with loss of weight and strength in association with continuous discomfort often results in a profound emotional deterioration, increasing the difficulties of patient care.

A number of mechanisms, either singly or in combination, may be responsible for the production of pain, including: (1) tumor infiltration and swelling of tissues enclosed in investing membranes that are richly supplied by sensory nerves, such as fascia or periosteum; (2) obstruction of a hollow viscus; (3) nerve compression by a tumor mass or by direct infiltration of the tumor into the nerves; (4) obstruction of blood vessels by pressure of a tumor mass or by infiltration into the vessel by tumor cells; and (5) reaction of the tissues surrounding the tumor, leading to inflammation, infection, and necrosis.

A considerable divergence of opinion exists regarding the information that should be given to the patient. At some point in their disease, most patients worry about the possibility of malignant disease, and many may avoid asking the physician directly since they do not wish to expose themselves to the truth. In some instances it is important for an individual to have full understanding of the nature of his illness so that he may have an opportunity to put his affairs in order. When this is not the case, there may be no advantage for the patient to be forced to face a grim prognosis. Many hospitals dealing largely with neoplastic diseases find it advisable to give almost

239

every patient a fairly straightforward explanation of his disease. While the patient is in the hospital and receiving active therapy, his morale may be surprisingly good, but after discharge a severe depression may occur and he looks forward to his doom with great mental anguish. Even when the patient is told that he is host to malignant disease, it is rarely necessary to offer a completely hopeless prognosis.

GENERAL PRINCIPLES

The expected duration of life and the site and severity of pain are the factors determining proper therapy. If life expectancy is less than three months, therapy is best limited to medications and blocks. Major surgical procedures ideally are reserved for patients who are more likely to benefit for a significant duration.

ANALGESICS

The use of nonnarcotic analgesics, such as the salicylates or the coal tar analgesics, is frequently of great benefit in the control of cancer pain. It is sometimes surprising to see patients with fairly advanced metastatic cancers doing well on aspirin. These nonaddictive drugs should be exploited to maximal use until more powerful medication becomes necessary.

Once the pain becomes demanding enough to require narcotics, some plan of action should be considered. If the life expectancy is less than three months, continued narcotic administration may be the management of choice. To defer as long as possible the problem of addiction, it is helpful to limit the use of any one narcotic to a three-week period, after which a new drug is administered. A change of narcotics is carried out even sooner than three weeks if the patient makes repeated demands for increased dosage. Rotation of drugs may help delay the onset of addiction but will not prevent it if narcotics are administered for a prolonged duration. When life expectancy is greater than three months, the management of choice is some method other than the use of narcotics.

RADIATION THERAPY AND CHEMOTHERAPY

X-ray therapy plays an ever increasing role in the management of pain associated with neoplasms. The object of radiation therapy is to damage tumor cells to the point at which mitosis is inhibited. Embryonal types of cells are damaged more quickly by radiotherapy than adult forms. The shorter the life cycle of a cell, the more radiosensitive it is. Response of tumors to radiation can be accurately determined histologically.

Nitrogen mustard and its chemical analogues are standard chemotherapeutic agents for the management of lymphomas and allied neoplasms. These drugs interfere with the utilization of nucleic acids in the malignant cells and impair the processes of abnormal cell multiplication—the basis of malignant disease. If there is a key to cancer, it probably lies in the direction of chemo-therapy.

ENDOCRINES AND CANCER

The effects of estrogens and androgens on carcinoma of the prostate and carcinoma of the breast may be useful in the management of pain secondary to these neoplasms.

Treatment of *prostatic carcinoma* by castration combined with estrogen therapy is standard procedure and has been clearly demonstrated to have a beneficial effect on longevity if instituted before metastasis has occurred. Individuals who already have had metastases frequently obtain considerable relief from this form of therapy even though their survival time is not statistically prolonged. In favorable responses, the size of the primary lesion in the prostate may decrease, there may be a striking disappearance of pain, and occasionally there is x-ray evidence of diminution of bony metastases particularly in the pelvis and spine. By causing a decrease in androgens, the estrogens alter the environment of the tumor to such an extent that its growth is hampered significantly. After a variable period of improvement, a relapse usually sets in after which the patient is not likely to survive more than nine months, although he may derive relief of pain from retreatment with estrogens. Total bilateral adrenalectomy has been recommended by some investigators when other forms of therapy for prostatic carcinoma have ceased to be effective. The role this major surgery plays in the treatment of neoplastic disease has not yet been established.

Estrogen can be administered by the subcutaneous implantation of estradiol pellets (two 25 mg. pellets implanted at three-month intervals). It can also be administered intramuscularly as diethylstilbestrol in daily 3 mg. doses for three weeks followed by an oral maintenance dosage of 0.5 mg. three times daily.

Carcinoma of the breast is also affected by endocrine therapy. Oophorectomy is a standard procedure for all women with breast cancer prior to the menopause and for a five-year period thereafter. After failure of oophorectomy, androgens should be used. Younger patients are considered the most suitable for androgenic hormone therapy, but androgens may be given a trial for intractable pain problems due to breast cancer at any age. As in prostatic carcinoma, evidence of objective improvement can be demonstrated occasionally by a decrease in size of the local breast lesion and in metastases to bone. Subjective effects of this therapy are more common, such as relief of pain, a feeling of well being, increased appetite, and sometimes gain in weight. The disadvantage of androgen therapy is that it causes masculinization with hirsutism, enlargement of the clitoris, lowering of the pitch of the voice, and sometimes cutaneous edema and acne. The exact action of this hormone on breast cancer is not understood, but there is some speculation that it may be related to the effect of androgens on calcium metabolism.

The dosage of testosterone propionate is 50 to 100 mg. given intramuscularly three times weekly. Treatment should be continued for about ten weeks before considering abandonment if results are not obtained.

Estrogen therapy is also of great value in the management of patients with breast cancer. Patients who are at least five years beyond the menopause respond much more favorably to this hormone than younger individuals. The rare male who develops carcinoma of the breast also responds well to estrogens. The mechanism of action is unknown. The dosage of diethylstilbestrol is 5 mg. three times daily for several months, depending upon the reaction to the drug. In some refractory cases combined androgen-estrogen therapy has been effective.

Adrenalectomy and hypophysectomy have been advocated by some investigators for cancer of the breast, but these are not standard procedures.

REGIONAL PAIN CONTROL

The management of pain associated with neoplasms, which may involve any area of the body, requires an understanding of the techniques and procedures available for the control of pain in a specific region.

Scalp Pain

Neoplasms involving the scalp are not a frequent source of discomfort, and when pain is a problem it usually can be controlled by radiation therapy. Rarely intractable pain that does not respond to irradiation may occur in association with such a lesion. Procaine infiltration of the somatic nerves innervating the involved portions of scalp should be carried out. To obtain relief of pain it is usually necessary to block several nerves because of the overlap in sensory fields. Temporary pain relief following procaine infiltration is an indication for alcohol block of the identical nerves (Fig. 160).

Face Pain

Most malignant tumors that cause facial pain involve deep lying structures that receive their sensory innervation from many branches of the cranial nerves, and this makes treatment difficult. Infrequently superficial facial pain is seen when the cancer is confined to the skin of the face. Blocking the nerves innervating the painful area is easily carried out and is usually quite effective in these cases.

Cancer involving the orbit and its contents may be the cause of severe pain. The tumor usually involves the eye and is associated with blindness. In such cases, exenteration of the orbital cavity followed by radiation therapy is the treatment of choice and usually alleviates the pain. If pain persists, a total retrogasserian neurectomy usually results in symptomatic relief if pain is confined to the orbit. Occasionally, however, tumors in this position extend beyond the orbital confines to the maxillary antrum and the base of

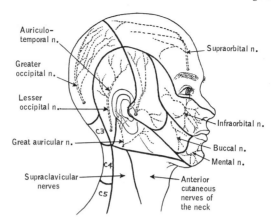

Figure 160. Peripheral nerve sensory fields of the scalp and face.

the skull. This extension may produce deep facial pain, upper jaw pain, and occasionally pain extending into the ear and upper cervical region. Widespread pain of this nature is not relieved by trigeminal surgery, and if all else fails, prefrontal lobotomy may be considered.

Cancer involving the maxillary antrum and upper jaw does not usually present a problem in pain management until the lesion is well advanced with widespread extension of the tumor. Pain from this condition is often circumscribed within the second or third division of the trigeminal nerve. Symptomatic relief may be derived from alcohol injection of the second or third division. Although trigeminal root section is a more certain method of interrupting these nerves, major surgery of this nature may not be tolerated by a debilitated patient with far advanced carcinoma.

Lower Jaw, Mouth, and Throat Pain

Cancer involving the lower jaw is invariably associated with severe pain. The extensive dosage of x-ray may cause radiation necrosis of the mandible, which produces severe burning pain. If the pain is unilateral, a block of the third division of the trigeminal nerve often results in symptomatic improvement. Frequently this condition causes bilateral lower jaw pain requiring bilateral sensory denervation of the jaw. Since a bilateral third division block would produce total paralysis of the muscles of mastication, it is necessary to block at least one side peripheral to the motor root. The inferior alveolar nerve, which is the sensory nerve to the mandible and lower lip, and the lingual nerve, which supplies sensation to the anterior two-thirds of the tongue and floor of the mouth, can be blocked with the same injection.

Technique of Inferior Alveolar and Lingual Nerve Block. This block is used routinely by dentists and can be performed easily (Fig. 161). The patient's jaw is opened widely, and the anterior border of the ramus of the mandible is prepared with aqueous Zephiran. A 4-inch, 22-gauge needle is introduced one-half inch above the last molar tooth until the bone of the anterior portion of the ramus is contacted; the needle is angled so that the shaft

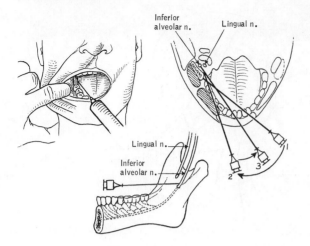

Figure 161. Technique of inferior alveolar and lingual nerve block.

is above the canine tooth on the side opposite the injection. Once bone is contacted, the shaft of the needle is swung laterally until it is parallel with the teeth on the same side, and the point is advanced slowly until it extends beyond the medial border of the ramus. The needle is then swung medially again until the shaft is above the first incisor of the same side, and the point is advanced a half inch. This should place the needle at the mandibular foramen. Injection of 2 cc. of alcohol will produce anesthesia of the inferior alveolar and lingual nerves.

The problem of pain control becomes increasingly difficult when the neoplasm extends to deeper structures. Involvement of the pharynx and the base of the tongue is extremely painful, swallowing becoming such an uncomfortably difficult process that the patient refrains from eating. In addition to the fifth cranial nerve, block or section of the glossopharyngeal nerve may be necessary. In some refractory cases surgical section of the fifth, ninth, and tenth cranial nerves and an upper cervical rhizotomy will not completely control the pain. Extensive cranial nerve sections of this nature should only be considered for unilateral pain. When the pain is bilateral, prefrontal lobotomy is probably a better choice.

Neck Pain

In a large number of cases malignant neoplasms metastasize or extend to the cervical lymph nodes. In spite of radical neck surgery and irradiation directed to this mass of neoplastic glands, intractable pain may persist. A posterior cervical rhizotomy is usually a most satisfactory procedure for control of pain in this region. A laminectomy is carried out by removing the arch of the atlas and the second and third cervical nerve roots. Section of the second, third, and fourth posterior roots on the side of the pain, or bilaterally if necessary, provides symptomatic relief. When the patient is too debilitated to tolerate surgery of this magnitude, an alcohol block of the cervical nerves may be given a trial.

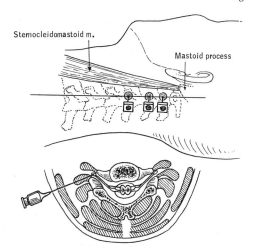

Figure 162. Technique of cervical nerve root block.

Technique of Cervical Nerve Root Block. The patient is placed in a supine position with a small pillow beneath the upper thoracic vertebrae to afford moderate extension, and the head is rotated toward the opposite side (Fig. 162). Rotation of the head displaces the sternocleidomastoid muscle and the carotid vessels anteriorly, bringing the transverse processes into a more superficial position. The transverse process of the sixth cervical vertebra (Chassaignac's tubercle) is quite prominent and easily palpated. A line drawn from Chassaignac's tubercle to a point one-half inch posterior to the mastoid tubercle identifies the level of the cervical transverse processes.

A skin wheal is made one fingerbreadth caudad to the mastoid process, on the line previously drawn, to overlie the second cervical transverse process. Two more wheals on the same line, separated from each other by a fingerbreadth, will overlie the third and fourth cervical transverse processes. A 2-inch, 22-gauge needle with a depth marker set at an inch and a half is advanced slowly through the first wheal perpendicular to the skin until contact is made with the transverse process of the second cervical vertebra. If the transverse process is not contacted at a depth of an inch and a half, the needle is partially withdrawn and redirected. It is important to avoid too deep an insertion of the needle, for if it passes anteriorly to the transverse process, it may enter the vertebral artery, or if between the transverse processes, it may perforate the dura and damage the cervical cord. Second and third needles are advanced through the second and third wheals in a similar fashion. When the needle placement is satisfactory, aspiration is performed to rule out perforation of a blood vessel or the subarachnoid space. Three cubic centimeters of a local anesthetic solution should produce a zone of anesthesia of the anterior and lateral cervical region and the suboccipital region. This can be followed by 2 cc. of alcohol injected through each needle.

Upper Extremity Pain

Upper extremity pain frequently occurs with several types of cancers. Bronchogenic carcinoma involving the apex of the lung (Pancoast tumor), cancer of the breast, and metastatic tumors involving the cervical vertebrae are among the most frequent neoplasms that produce pain in the upper limb. Management of pain in this region is technically difficult and remains a vexing problem.

Deafferentation of the upper extremity by means of an extensive posterior root section (posterior rhizotomy) may often relieve the pain but almost invariably results in a flail-like, numb upper limb, which is useless and a source of considerable difficulty and annoyance to the patient. This complication has discouraged widespread use of the procedure for control of upper extremity pain.

Anterolateral cordotomy, if performed at the first cervical segment, may produce a zone of sensory anesthesia above the involved limb and be effective in controlling pain. This procedure is technically difficult, and often the generally poor condition of the patient and a limited life expectancy may contraindicate such major surgery.

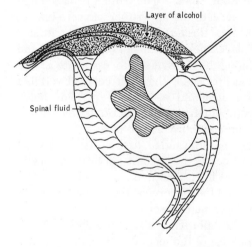

Figure 163. Diagram illustrating layering of the hypobaric alcohol injected into the subarachnoid space to affect the uppermost nerve roots.

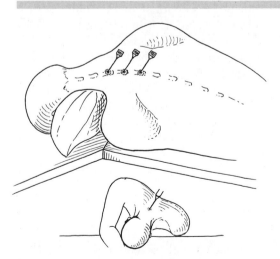

Figure 164. Technique of lower cervical and upper thoracic subarachnoid alcohol block.

Prefrontal lobotomy is considered by some to be the procedure of choice because of the technical difficulties and complications associated with the two procedures just discussed. When the patient's condition is such that high cervical cordotomy would not be tolerated, a subarachnoid alcohol injection should be given a trial before considering lobotomy. This is a potentially dangerous method of management, yet in view of the alternative, it should be considered in selected cases.

Technique of Subarachnoid Alcohol Block. Absolute ethyl alcohol, a neurolytic agent that destroys nerve fibers, is hypobaric, having a specific gravity much less than that of spinal fluid. Subarachnoid alcohol block technique is based upon this property of the alcohol, which when slowly injected into the cerebrospinal fluid forms a layer on top of the spinal fluid. If the patient is positioned properly at the time of the injection, the agent will bathe the nerve roots in a specific area and destroy the thin myelinated and unmyelinated pain fibers (Fig. 163). The obvious problem associated with this technique is the necessity for limiting the effects of the alcohol to the desired segment of the spinal cord and avoiding excessive spread or "spill-over" of the alcohol.

Because of the importance of maintaining the patient in the proper position for an hour following the injection, this procedure should always be performed with a nurse in constant attendance who is aware of the possible complications. It is imperative that the patient be watched carefully for this period of time, since prolonged maintenance of any position eventually becomes irksome and uncomfortable and leads to potentially dangerous shifting of the body if the patient is left unwatched. This is more likely to occur when the patient is severely debilitated and emotionally deteriorated by the chronic pain of cancer. A full discussion of the procedure, including the potential complications, should be given the patient and family, and the physician should stress that it may be necessary to repeat the block several times to achieve satisfactory relief of pain.

The procedure is best performed on an operating table because of the ease with which the table can be manipulated to various positions. For a block affecting the upper extremity, the patient is placed in a semilateral position with the side to be blocked uppermost. Pillows are placed beneath the upper chest and neck, creating a curvature of the cervical spine to make the lower cervical and upper thoracic spine the highest point in the spinal curve (Fig. 164). The cervical interspaces are often difficult to palpate, but the midline is easily ascertained, and a fairly reliable approximation of interspaces can be made by using the prominent spinous process of C7 as a guide. A 20-gauge, short, beveled spinal needle is introduced through the C5-C6 interspace with great care, millimeter by millimeter. Penetration of the dura is usually indicated by the typical sensation of perforating a parchment-like layer. Occasionally this usual "snap" is absent, and it is necessary to withdraw the stylet and gently aspirate the needle at frequent intervals. Aspiration may be necessary because occasionally the pressure of the spinal fluid may be so low that fluid does not appear spontaneously at the hub of the needle. Once the free flow of spinal fluid indicates entrance into the subarachnoid space, advancement of the needle is halted to avoid insertion

247

of the needle point into the substance of the spinal cord. Inadvertent injection of alcohol into the cord substance will produce quadriplegia.

After proper placement of the first needle, the same technique is used to insert needles between the C6-C7 and C7-T1 interspaces. Greater effectiveness follows the injection of small amounts of alcohol through several needles rather than injection of a larger quantity of alcohol through a single needle in an effort to obtain a widespread block. The multiple needle technique also minimizes the excessive spread or "spillover" of alcohol, since a small amount is more quickly fixed within the area of the needle and the effects are likely to remain confined to the injected segment. A 1 cc. tuberculin syringe is used to inject 0.25 cc. of absolute alcohol very slowly through each needle, taking a full minute to inject each 0.1 cc. After completion of the injection through one needle, the stylet is replaced and the injection is repeated through the next needle.

While the injection is proceeding, the patient is constantly tested with a sharp pin to determine the extent of hypesthesia. If the effect of this initial injection appears inadequate, the quantity can be increased to a total of 0.75 cc. through each needle. It is safer to repeat the injection later than to exceed this quantity during a single session. The blood pressure, pulse, and general status are recorded for an hour following the injection. After an hour has elapsed, the needles are removed. The patient is then maintained in a supine position with the bed in slight head-down position for 24 hours. At the end of 24 hours the patient is allowed out of bed.

The results of the block are usually realized immediately after the injection, but occasionally the full effect does not occur until several days following the injection. For this reason it is advisable to wait for four or five days before repeating the block. When relief of pain is achieved, it usually lasts about three months. This block may involve the anterior roots in the cervical region, causing weakness of the involved extremity. This is usually acceptable to the patient, since use of the limb is severely hampered by the original pain. Another complication of this procedure is spinal cord damage caused either by direct trauma of the needle or the reaction to the alcohol. Spinal cord symptoms may vary from transient sphincter weakness to complete quadriplegia. A rare complication of this procedure may occur when through misunderstanding or inability of the patient to cooperate, the head is elevated precipitously. This may allow the hypobaric alcohol to rise and affect the vital cerebral centers. Respiratory and circulatory collapse may occur and lead to death.

A recently developed technique of subarachnoid injection using phenol crystals dissolved in Pantopaque may have certain advantages over alcohol. The phenol-Pantopaque mixture is radiopaque; hence, it can be positioned accurately under fluoroscopic guidance as in the technique used in myelography. Preliminary reports of this method indicate considerable promise.

Chest Pain

The parenchyma of the lung and its visceral pleura are insensitive to pain so that neoplastic disease causing pain in the chest indicates spread of the lesion to the parietal pleura or involvement of the main bronchi and trachea. When the pain involves a limited segment of the chest wall, posterior rhizotomy, which produces anesthesia in the involved area, usually gives symptomatic relief. For pain that is more diffuse it may be necessary to consider spinothalamic cordotomy, although it may be technically difficult to achieve a high enough level of hypesthesia to provide pain relief. When the patient is too debilitated to tolerate surgery, segmental subarachnoid block may be indicated. A significant technical problem is the difficulty of performing a subarachnoid tap in the thoracic region because of the frequent overlap of the spinous processes and laminae.

Abdominal and Pelvic Pain

Intractable pain in the abdomen and pelvis frequently occurs in association with malignant disease. In such situations that cannot be controlled with

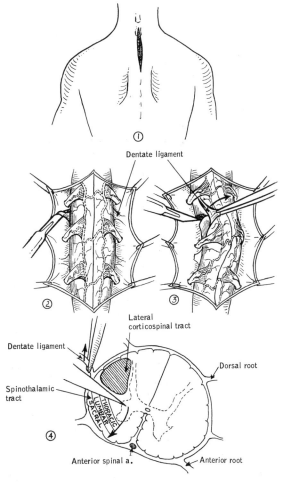

Figure 165. Technique of spinothalamic cordotomy. (1) Incision. (2) Cutting dentate ligament. (3) Incision into cord. (4) Diagrammatic cross section of cord incision.

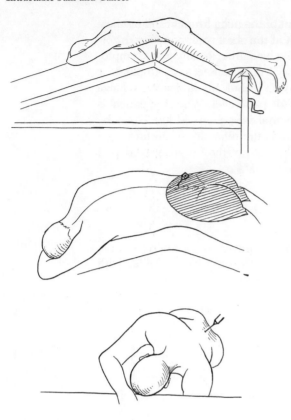

Figure 166. Lumbosacral subarachnoid alcohol block to produce saddle anesthesia. A hospital bed can be used to position the patient.

medication, spinothalamic cordotomy is the procedure of choice. The excellent results of this operation, when performed for pain located below the costal margin, have made it a standard procedure in neurosurgical practice.

Technique of Cordotomy. Cordotomy is often carried out under local anesthesia to assure an adequate level of sensory anesthesia at the time of surgery; an assistant can test for pain sensation with a pin immediately after the incision is made into the cord (Fig. 165). If the level is inadequate, the extent of the incision can be increased. My experience with local anesthesia has not been particularly fruitful, for sensory levels obtained at surgery from uncooperative and restless patients are often misleading, and therefore endothracheal anesthesia is used routinely in our clinic. The usual midline incision is made to expose the first three thoracic vertebrae. A laminectomy is carried out, removing the spines and laminae of T2 and T3. The dura is opened in the midline and tacked laterally to the muscles for retraction. The dentate ligaments are sectioned to permit rotation of the cord. The cord is rotated and a number 11 blade is inserted a measured depth of 4.5 mm. at the site of attachment of the dentate ligament to the cord. The knife blade is rotated anteriorly to incise the anterior quadrant of the cord, taking care to avoid injury to the anterior spinal artery. When bilateral cordotomy is performed, the incisions are spaced at least one segment apart. Laminectomy closure is performed in the usual fashion.

Frequently, advanced pelvic cancers produce pain that is limited to the perineum and cause weakness of the sphincter. This problem often can be managed easily by subarachnoid alcohol injection in the lumbosacral region. The needle is introduced in the L5 and S1 interspace with the patient prone in a hips-up, head-down position. One cubic centimeter of absolute alcohol is used with the usual precautions (Fig. 166).

Index

Date Due

Dec 15			
FEB 25 '72			
~~APR 15 '72~~			
May 10			
Nov 30 '72			
Mar 20 '73			
Nov 25 '73			
~~Apr 25 '74~~			
Aug 1 75			
DEC 15 '76			
DEC 1 '78			
MAR 16 '82			
MAR 15 1984			